HEALING MUDRAS
For Your MIND

VOLUME II.

NEW REVISED
FULL COLOR EDITION

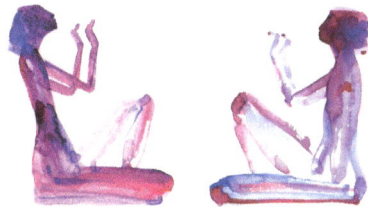

SABRINA MESKO Ph.D.H.

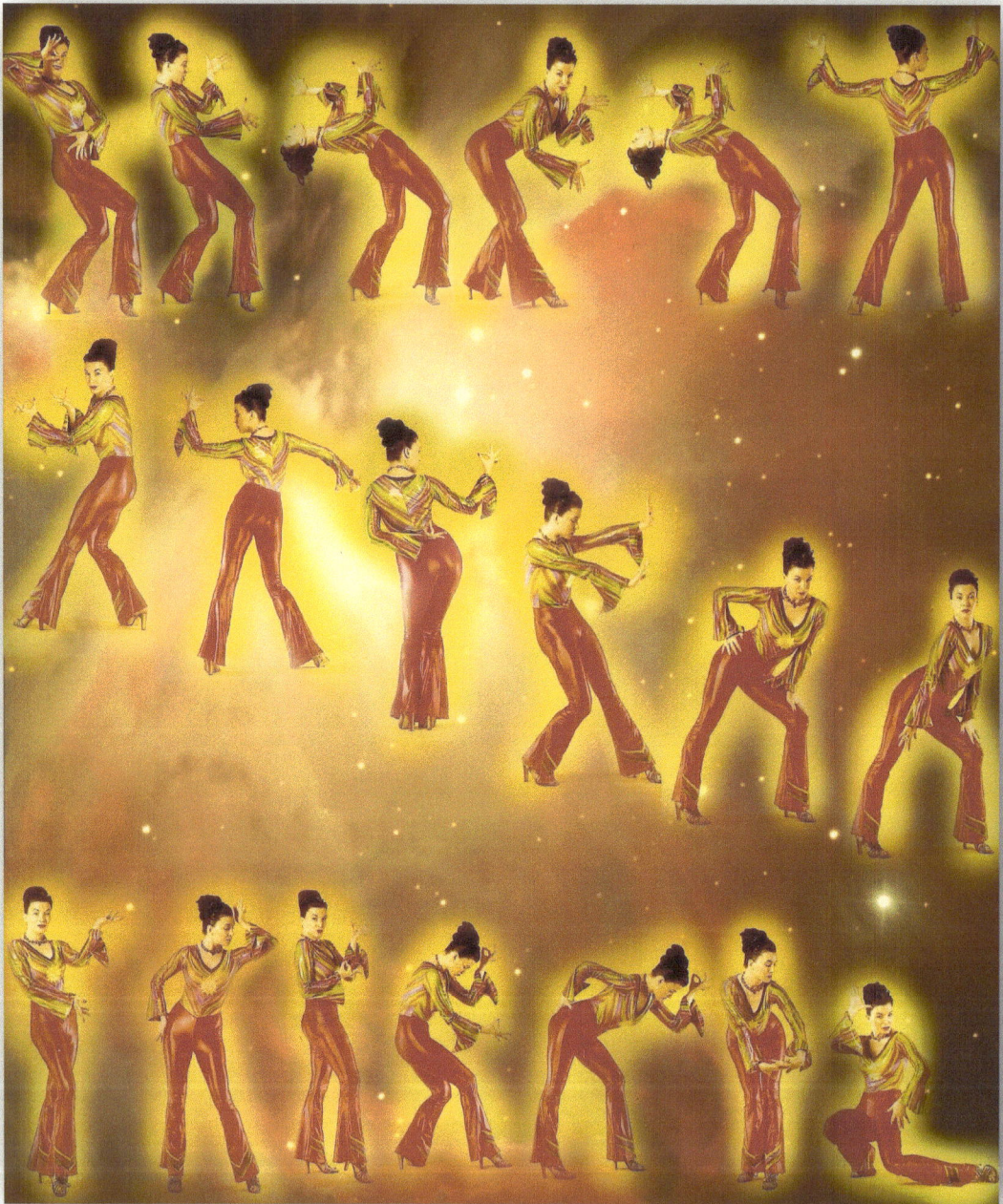

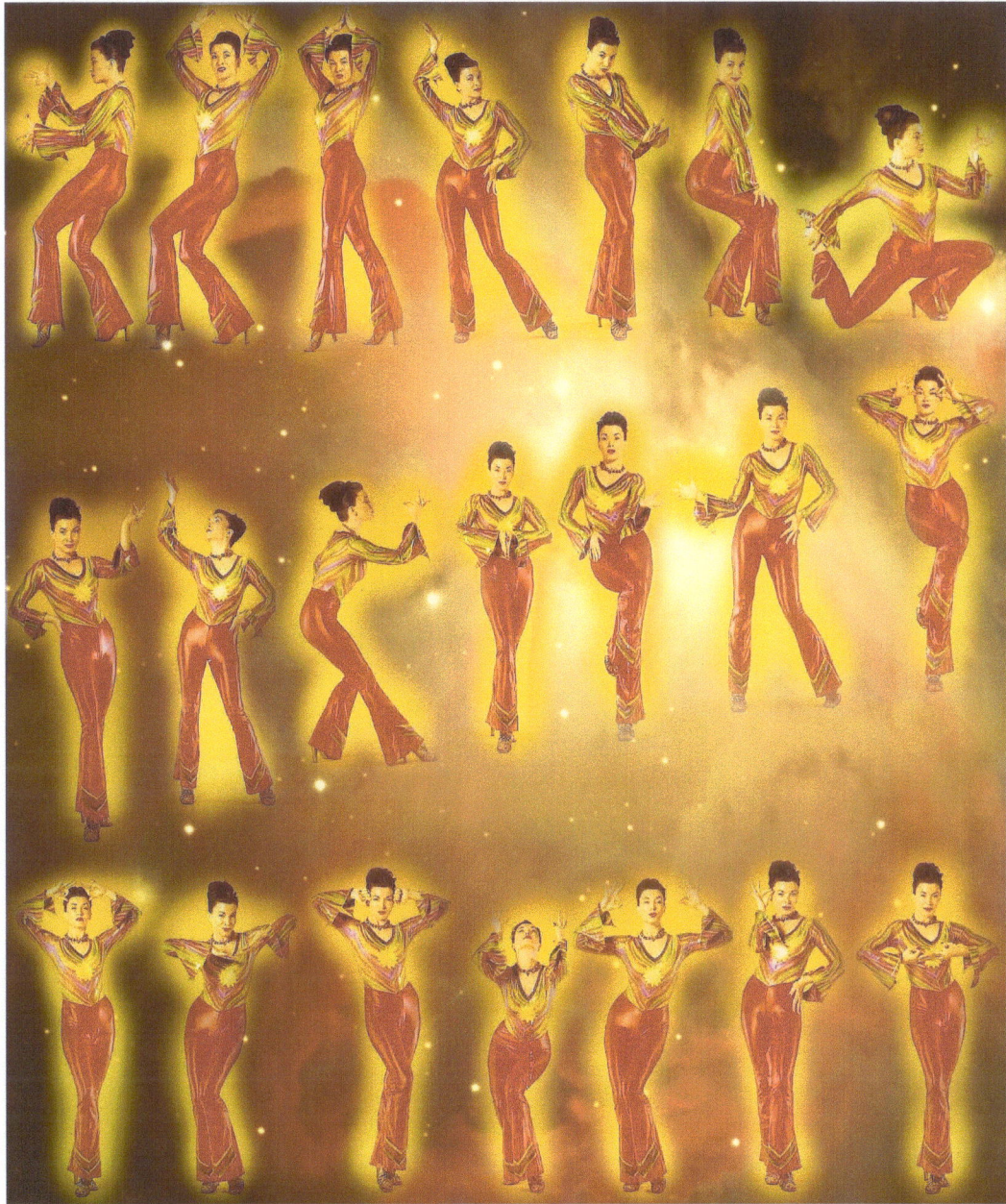

The material contained in this book is not intended as medical advice.
If you have a medical issue or illness, consult a qualified physician.

A Mudra Hands™ Book
Published by Mudra Hands Publishing

Photography by Dorothy Low
Illustrations by Kiar Mesko
Costume design, photo design, and styling by Sabrina Mesko
Cover photo by Dorothy Low
On The Cover ~ MUDRA for Facing Fear

Printed in the United States of America

ISBN-13: 978-0615811475
ISBN-10: 0615811477

Originally published by Random House in 2000
Under the title *Healing Mudras -Yoga for Your Hands*
New, revised, updated and expanded

To the greatest parents in the world,
Bibi and Kiar

By SABRINA MESKO

HEALING MUDRAS
Yoga for Your Hands
Random House - Original edition

POWER MUDRAS
Yoga Hand Postures for Women
Random House - Original edition

MUDRA - GESTURES OF POWER
DVD - Sounds True

CHAKRA MUDRAS DVD set
HAND YOGA for Vitality, Creativity and Success
HAND YOGA for Concentration, Love and Longevity

HEALING MUDRAS
Yoga for Your Hands - New Edition

HEALING MUDRAS - New Edition in full color:
Healing Mudras I. ~ For Your Body
Healing Mudras II. ~ For Your Mind
Healing Mudras III. ~ For Your Soul

POWER MUDRAS
Yoga Hand Postures for Women - New Edition

MUDRA THERAPY
Hand Yoga for Pain Management and Conquering Illness

YOGA MIND
45 Meditations for Inner Peace, Prosperity and Protection

MUDRAS for ASTROLOGICAL SIGNS
Volumes I. ~ XII.

MUDRAS for ARIES, TAURUS, GEMINI, CANCER, LEO, VIRGO, LIBRA, SCORPIO, SAGITTARIUS, CAPRICORN, AQUARIUS, PISCES
12 Book Series

LOVE MUDRAS
Hand Yoga for Two

MUDRAS AND CRYSTALS
The Alchemy of Energy Protection

INTERNATIONAL BESTSELLER

HEALING MUDRAS

For Your

MIND

SABRINA MESKO
VOLUME II.

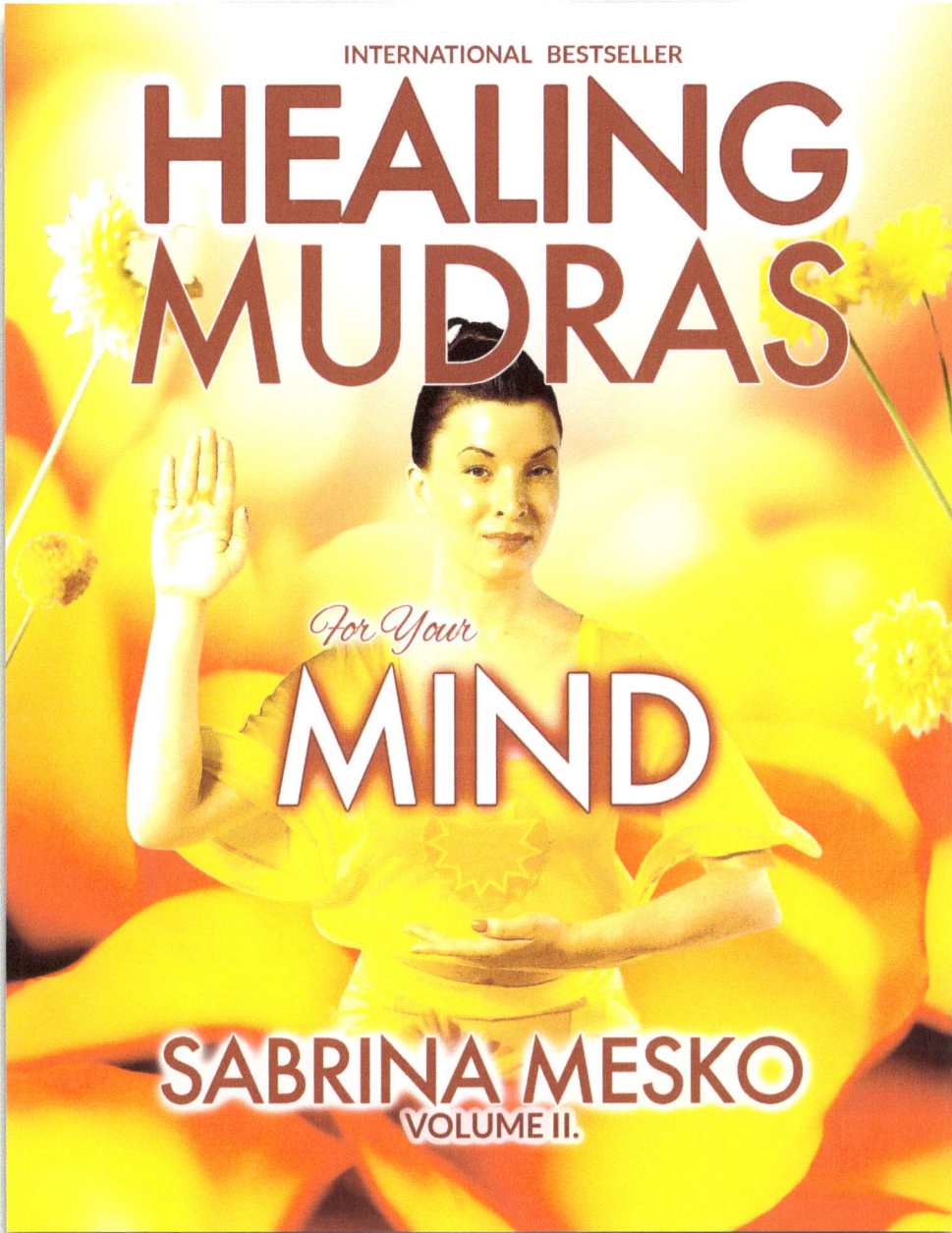

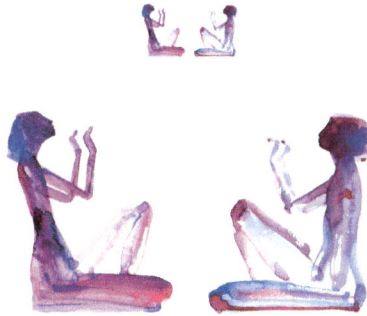

CONTENTS

MUDRAS FOR YOUR MIND

HEALING MUDRAS
FOR
YOUR MIND

YOGA FOR YOUR HANDS

INTRODUCTION

Mudras are the ancient sacred codes to your body, mind and spirit. They are a part of your everyday lives, intuitively used and intricately affecting your energy level, self-healing capacity and energy reception and output. The healing powers of Mudras are undeniable and needed now more than ever.

Thirteen years have passed since the original HEALING MUDRAS was published. As every author will tell you, the moment you let the book out of your hands, it begins a life of its own. Whether it is a long life or a short one, it depends on so many factors. HEALING MUDRAS is long-lived, for it has been translated into over 14 languages and has positively affected thousands of Mudra practitioners around the world. Since the first publication, I have traveled the globe, taught people these powerful ancient techniques in different languages, and received countless letters of gratitude for bringing Mudras into today's spotlight. Every time I receive a reader's letter, I am deeply joyful that another person has benefited from these techniques, and humbled for the opportunity of being a part of that process. I am only the messenger and instrument to convey these ancient sacred Mudras. It is truly a part of my life's mission and an honor to have had the pleasure of teaching Mudras to all kinds of audiences, all ages, all cultures, religions and spiritual convictions, or openness to healing aspects of such practices. I can honestly say that each and every person who practiced Mudras, has experienced the power magnitude of positive effects. It has been an amazing journey that continues to this day.

Mudras will always be a profound part of my life, and since the readers have asked me numerous times when my next project will be released, I have created a double DVD series titled Chakra Mudras to help expand available practice materials. And now the time has come for an updated NEW edition HEALING MUDRAS - a new revised version of the first book with the additional chapter. I have decided to offer the reader two choices; a complete book with black and white photographs, and a color version of the book in three separate volumes, for Body, Mind and Soul. The color edition was my original wish for the look and feel of the book and is now realized. What you hold in your hands is the Volume II. with full color photographs, nevertheless you, my dear reader, have the choice.

Thru the years passed I have often reflected on my destined meeting with my teacher Yogi Bhajan. I remain eternally grateful for everything he taught me and continue to follow every detail of his personal Mudra practice and teaching instructions.

My early years as a professional ballerina left within me a permanent imprint of discipline and persistence and I apply that to every aspect of my work with Mudras. They are such precise and intricate hand positions that need to be practiced with accuracy and focus to produce optimal results. You have to be present, truly immerse yourself into the Mudra practice and then....most wondrous things happen. Mudras take charge and you can follow your hands and experience the true depth of these ancient codes. Suddenly your soul power unlocks and is set free, your life perspective changes and you understand and perceive this earthly experience in a deeper, more profound way, all the while with a healthy distance from challenging times and expanded understanding of fortunate ones.

Each lifetime seems to have a hidden pendulum that swings back and forth, it seems there is an invisible balance that remains, no matter how it all appears to others from the outside. There is an order, there is a purpose and there is a designated path that each one of us is on, but all of our life's mysteries cannot be revealed at once. We must remain attentive in the present, the now, to truly experience every nuance that this earthly incarnation offers to teach us. If we understand and respect the pendulum, the balance will remain intact. If we fight it, it will be thrown off.

The inner balance is the true key to be able to journey thru life with enduring vigor and loving generosity while surrendering the final outcome to the invisible universal power that resides in us all. We must trust this universal navigation, for it knows us better than we ever will. It loves us more than we ever will. And it has a better plan for us than we could ever imagine. Mudras are one of these sacred keys, for they are connected to your every move and every breath. Understand them, use them, and let them serve you on your way to enlightenment, self-realization, healing, and the absolute fulfillment of your optimal potential.

As always, I remain eternally grateful for being given the opportunity to be the instrument for the transmission of these sacred teachings to you.

One in Spirit, love, and Peace. Blessings to all,

Sabrina

The History and Art of MUDRA

Hand gestures have been native to every culture on earth and can be seen as intrinsic to civilization: Ancient Egyptians, Romans, Greeks, Persians, Aborigines in Australia, ancient Indians and Chinese, Africans, Turks, Fijians, Mayan cultures, Inuit, and the Native American nations all used hand gestures.

Today, we still use hand language. Think about the universal handshake – a sign of friendship and peace. Applause is the language for approval and enthusiasm; the pointed index finger is used to scold; an upraised hand with the palm -out signals us to stop.

There are many points of view regarding the development of hand gestures. Scientists have proved that even apes communicate with their hands and firmly believe that hand gestures were basis for speech. A blind child who has never been able to see will still clap his hands to express excitement and happiness. Many hand gestures are universal, dating back thousands of years. In Egypt almost five thousand years ago, hand gestures were performed in prayer rituals by high priests and priestesses. Sacred hand gestures were key to communicating with the gods, manifesting miracles, and connecting with the afterlife. Egyptians carved these sacred gestures in bas-reliefs on the walls of and inside the pyramids, and they became the basis for their hieroglyphs. From Egypt these movements and knowledge of their spiritual power and usage traveled to India and Greece.

In India, these gestures were named "mudras," a Sanskrit word, and they became an irreplaceable part of yoga, which aimed to connect the practitioner to divine and cosmic energy. Mudras became the essence of this divine communication in Buddhism and Hinduism. Buddhist priests developed the understanding of mudras still further and used them to close prayer rituals, a practice that has remained alive to this day.

Plato placed hand gestures among the civil virtues in ancient Greece, where there was a distinct classification of hand gestures into comic, tragic, and satiric. From Egypt and Greece, these hand gestures were brought to Rome, where they became intrinsic to popular discourse and culture.

In the reign of Emperor Augustus in Rome, performances of hand gestures in pantomimic dances were a great personal delight of the emperor. Competitions were held between the best hand – gesture dancers, and all Rome was split into factions about their favorites. The most distinguished performer was often called the Dancing Philosopher.

In the year 190, there were six thousand performers in Rome devoted to the art of hand gesture. Their popularity continued until the sixth century A.D. Sacred hand gestures were also used in religious practice among Jews. In various portrayals of Moses we can observe him using mudras with gestures of blessing, divine protection, knowledge, and receiving guidance from the divine.

In Christianity, mudras took on a less noticeable form. Stylized hand poses are almost always present in portrayals of Jesus, but most people were not taught the significance of these poses. So the people in Western cultures lost the awareness of the healing and sacred power of the mudras and used them more as expressive communication gestures.

In Italian paintings before and during the renaissance, one of the most common hand poses is that of the connected thumb and index finger. Its meaning is that the ego – the index finger – is bowing to God – the thumb – in love and unity. In popular Neapolitan use, that gesture is called the kissing of the thumb and finger – the sign of love. In secular portraits, that gesture translates into approval of love and marriage. Some Native Americans also used that hand gesture when indicating that they thought something was good and approved of it.

Another common gesture in religious paintings is that of the palm turned upward. This pose dates back centuries and signifies openness and inquiry. In this book, it is part of the mudra of asking for guidance, and it has a part in mudra for facing fear. When you ask the Universe to protect and guide you, the palm is held so that something can be placed in your hand – something can come to you. American Indians translated this gesture into: Give me!

A gesture in which the pointed index finger moves in a circle has a universal connection – specifically, "no" – rejection in Italian, native American, and Japanese cultures, among others. When the index finger is pointed but motionless in popular usage and in high Italian art, it means indication, justice, pointing something out (which has led to the actual name of index for the forefinger). It can also mean silence, attention, number, mediation, and demonstration. Native Americans were among the most famed hand – sign communicators, usually signing in front of strangers. Early white settles actually believed that the American Indians rarely used spoken language, since the settlers most often saw them using hand gestures that Europeans didn't understand. Later on, Native Americans would play a key role in communicating with hearing – impaired children.

In Mexico, hand signs are found in elaborate ancient carvings, and they are also painted on ancient Greek and Homeric vases and pottery writings. The Chinese alphabet actually originated as the depiction of hand gestures. There are many commonalities among the hand gestures of Native American, Chinese, Egyptian, and African cultures. I hope that archeologists, anthropologists, and linguists can eventually piece together how these universal gestures come to be used in such different parts of the world. Hand gestures are the mother of all communication and are supremely powerful. The art of mudra is divinely inspired: It enables us to communicate with the divine, develop and aspire to higher qualities, and keep a universally popular language. Mudra is our connection to the divine play of the cosmos.

The time has come to revive and appreciate the gift of mudras practice to utilize these efficient, powerful ancient techniques in your everyday life. Mudra can help you follow your dreams: Your life is in your hands. There are no limitations.

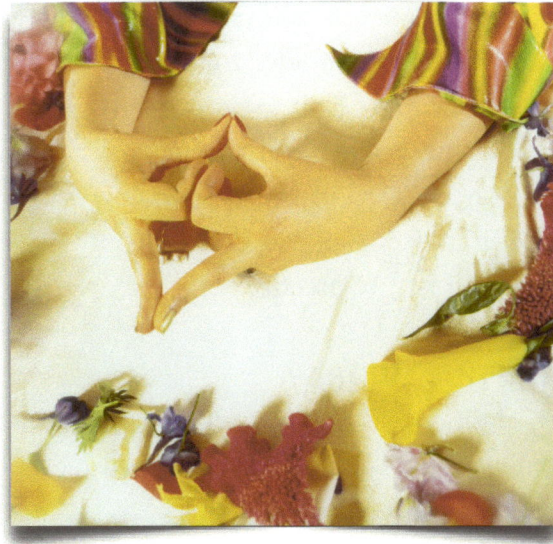

MUDRA FOR TRANQUILIZING YOUR MIND

THE PRACTICE OF MUDRA

INSTRUCTIONS FOR PRACTICE

WHERE DO I PRACTICE MUDRA?

To practice mudra, find a quiet, peaceful, and private place where no one can disturb you. If that is not always possible, you can usually practice most of the mudras that are unobtrusive just about anywhere.

HOW DO I PRACTICE MUDRA?

During the practice, it is best to sit in a comfortable position. You can sit on a pillow or blanket in a cross-legged position, or in a chair, but make sure your weight on both feet is equal. It is most important that you keep your back straight. Maintain a comfortable sitting posture that does *not* give you pain.

WHEN SHOULD I PRACTICE MUDRA?

You can practice a mudra virtually any time that you feel the need to connect with the energy that it gives you. If you are practicing a mudra for insight or to enhance your meditation, however, the easiest time to concentrate is in the morning right after you wake up or in the evening before going to sleep. You should never practice a mudra on a full stomach, because your body-mind's energy is concentrated in your abdomen. Your overall energy is slow and needs to be permitted to be unimpeded as it focuses on turning nourishment into physical energy. After a meal, wait an hour before practice.

HOW OFTEN CAN I PRACTICE MUDRA?

You can practice as many mudras a day as you wish, but to obtain the full benefit that a mudra can give you, you will want to establish at least one three - minute set time during the day in which to grow comfortable with your mudra.

To feel the benefits faster, I recommend that you practice the mudra twice a day, each time for at least three minutes. Select a mudra that addresses a problem you have or a quality you want to develop, and make it a point to practice that mudra every day.

HOW LONG SHOULD I PRACTICE A MUDRA?

Your should practice a mudra in the beginning for at least three minutes a day, but when you have built up your strength and ability to hold the mudra and evoke its energy, you can extend your practice to eleven minutes. Ultimately, you may want to build up your practice to thirty-one minutes a day.

Most of the mudras will give you immediate results, in the form of more energy, clarity and peace of mind, or insight. More challenging or entrenched problems, however, will require more discipline and perseverance in your practice. It will take a few weeks of practice for the mudra to come into full effect and help you feel a profound transformation that will eliminate or resolve your problem.

MEDITATION

There are many different meditative techniques. If you have not meditated before, the simplest way to begin meditating is to find a quiet place and sit comfortably. Bring your attention to your breath: Exhale and inhale slowly through your nose and concentrate on your breath as it travels in and out of your body. As you concentrate, allow the awareness of your breath to still your mind and relax your body. You have begun to experience the essential state of meditation.

Meditation will lower your body temperature, so, when you plan to meditate for longer than eleven minutes, you should cover your back and shoulders with a shawl before sitting down. With mudras and proper breathing, you can achieve deeper levels of meditation. You will experience peace, relaxation, rejuvenation, and higher levels of consciousness.

Your intuition, patience, and wisdom will increase greatly, as will your personal magnetism and level of energetic vibration.

BREATHING

Proper breathing is essential when practicing a mudra. There are basically two types of breathing:

In **LONG DEEP BREATHING**, you take your time inhaling and exhaling slowly and completely, through your nose.

When you inhale, relax your abdomen and expand the chest.

When exhaling, deflate the chest and pull in the stomach to help expel the air. This technique of breathing will help you relax, calm down, and be more patient.

In the **SHORT BREATH OF FIRE**, inhale and exhale through the nose at a much faster pace. Focus on your navel point, expanding for inhalation and contracting on exhalation. Both parts are equal in time and can be quite rapid: two to three breaths per second.

This technique has a more invigorating effect.

Both techniques are very cleansing and healing.

During your mudra practice, it is best to use Long Deep Breathing except where noted.

CONCENTRATION

While practicing any mudra it is important to concentrate on the energy center of your Third Eye, which is between your eyebrows. Your Third Eye is the point of your body-mind that connects most easily to the higher sources of energy within you and around you.

As you practice meditation and mudra, if your mind wonders, gently bring your attention back to your breath and your mudra. Breathe in and out. You will experience a very powerful effect, a heightening of energy, throughout your entire body. Mudra practice affects each individual differently at different times. Sometimes you may feel a slight tingling sensation in your hands and arms; at other times, you may experience a sudden rush of energy through our spine. Allow yourself to feel and notice whatever comes up for you. Concentrating on the different feelings, allowing them to be there, will magnify the healing benefits to your body, mind and spirit.

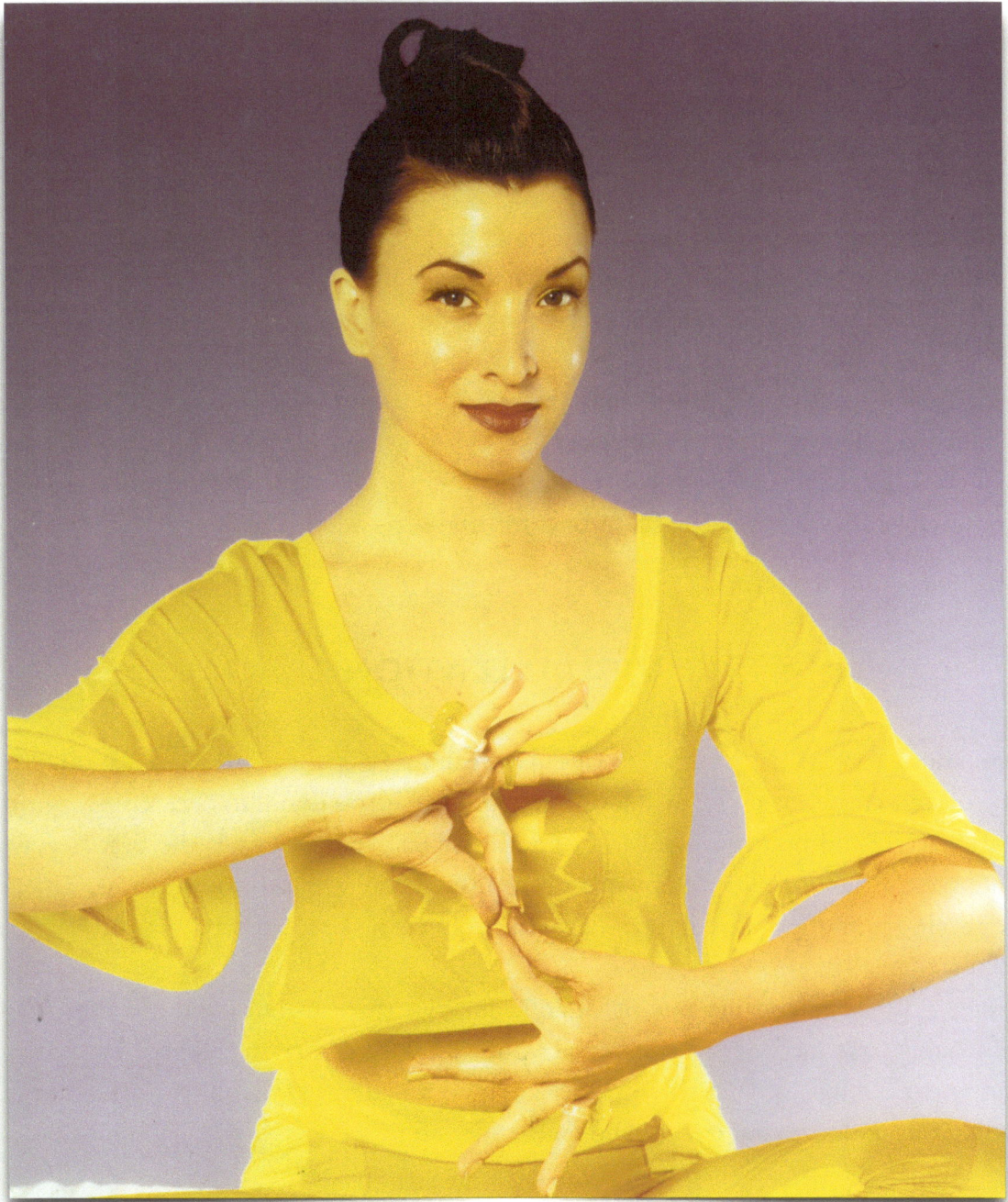

Your Third Eye center is the point between the eyebrows.
By focusing your mind's attention on this energy center of intuition,
you can practice visualization and receive guidance and visions.
It is your window to infinite possibilities.

EYE MOVEMENTS

The eyes are an important element in the practice of mudra. How you use them will increase your concentration.

You can keep them half open and gently direct them to look over the tip of your nose. Do not cross your eyes to do this. Just look down and slightly in so that you perceive the end of your nose. This is a very beneficial exercise for your eyesight.

Another practice is to close your eyelids and gently aim your eyes upward toward the area of the Third Eye. If you need to keep your eyes open as you meditate, look into the middle distance and relax the eyelids. Most important, the eye focus should always be done *gently*. Never force your eyes into a painful or uncomfortable position.

VISUALIZATION

We all know how to daydream. Actually daydreaming is a form of visualization. In your mind you can create a picture, world, or dream in which you desire to live. Visualizing where you want to be and how you want to live and manifest your energy is the first step toward making your dream a reality. Mudra practice can help you actualize your dreams. The power of your mind is limitless. Live it, breathe it, and you will make it a reality.

For example: While practicing a mudra for anti aging, visualize in your mind a healthy, youthful glow around your face. See yourself and your face vibrant and recharged. By adding the power of your mind to your daily practice of mudra and visualization, you will change and improve your outlook, your energy, and your entire life.

As another example, when practicing a mudra for insight, see yourself as having reached a happy solution for a problem you've been trying to resolve. Visualize how you would feel if your concern were over. From this visualization will emerge a positive approach to creating a good outcome.

POSITIVE AFFIRMATIONS AND PRAYER

When you meditate, your mind becomes fine-tuned to your body's needs and you gain in healing capacity. It is important before you meditate to make a positive affirmation for yourself. You can also affirm positive energy for another person, just as you would in a prayer.

Example: When practicing the mudra for dieting it is beneficial to affirm:
"I am eating only healthful food. I am healthy, trim, and full. I am sticking to my diet."
This simple affirmation will have a positive effect on you.

When meditating or praying for someone else, it is helpful to see them surrounded by white or violet light and affirm: "My friend is healthy, happy, full of life, and smiling."
Your affirmation should always be formed in the resent tense. "I am calm," not "I will be or want to be calm." or, "I see the solution in my meditation." This positive statement creates powerful energy vibrations. Your energy is sent out into the Universe and manifests your desires and intentions, enabling you to accomplish your goals successfully, honorably, and compassionately. Prayer and affirmations are especially powerful during the practice of mudra when your mind is calm and your concentration is magnified.

MANTRA

While you may prefer to practice your mudra and meditation using your affirmation, you may also want to try using a mantra. Mantras are ancient Sanskrit healing words that have a powerful effect on your entire being when chanted repeatedly during meditation or mudra practice. The hard palate in your mouth has fifty-eight energy points that connect to your entire body. Stimulating these points with sound vibrations affects your mental and physical energy. Certain sounds that stimulate these points have a very healing quality. When you repeat aloud or whisper these ancient mantras or scientific healing-sound combinations, the meridians on your hard palate are activated in a specific order that re-patterns the energy of your whole system. There are three basic mantras that you will find in this book in different combinations:

EK ONG KAR
One Creator, God Is One

SA TA NA MA
Infinity, Birth, Death, Rebirth

HAR HARE HAREE
WAHE GURU
Hah-rah; hah-ray; hah-ree; wa -hay; guh-roo
God is the Creator of Supreme Power and Wisdom

Not every mudra practice requires a mantra. All mudras can be practiced in silence to the rhythm of your breathing. You can use the mantras when you are struggling with a restless mind, since focusing on the words will help center you. Follow your intuition during the mudra practice and if you are drawn to chanting the mantras, try them when you feel it is right. You will experience profound peace, joy, and passion. Your soul will sing with the Universe.

THE MANTRA PRONUNCIATION GUIDE

A like *a* in about
AA like the *a* in want
AY like *ay* in say
AI like the *a* in sand
I like the *i* in bit
U like the *u* in put
OO like the *oo* in good
O like the *o* in no
E like the *ay* in say
EE like the *e* in meet
AAU like the *ow* in now
SAT rhymes with "what"
NAM rhymes with "mom"
WAHE – sounds like wa-hay
GU – sounds like "put"
Emphasize the"ch" at the end of every " such."Pronounce the consonant v softly.
Roll the *rs* slightly. When chanting the mantra like " Haree Har Haree Har,"
make sure you do not move your lips, and pronounce it with the tongue only.

THE HANDS

Both hands and all ten fingers have individual, distinct meanings. Each corresponds to the energy of a different body part and to the energy of our solar system. The right hand is influenced by the Sun and represents the male side of one's nature. The left hand is ruled by the Moon and represents the female aspect of one's nature.

The right hand is the receiver while the left is the giver of positive powers. These meanings are also reflected in the hand positions of mudras.
Each finger is associated with a special ability, tendency, or characteristic and how it affects your life.

The **THUMB** symbolizes God. When the rest of your fingers connect to the thumb you symbolically bow to God. The Thumb is associated with the planet Mars and represents willpower, logic, love, and ego. The angle it makes with the rest of your hand when relaxed indicates your character. A distance between the thumb and index fingers of around ninety degrees indicates you are generous, kindhearted, and giving. A distance of about sixty degrees suggests a logical, rational character. A thirty-degree space indicates a secretive, sensitive, and cautious person. A long, strong thumb reveals a strong personality, willpower, and the ability to change your destiny.
The **INDEX** finger is influenced by the planet Jupiter and represents your knowledge, wisdom, sense of power, and self-confidence.
The **MIDDLE** finger is the indicator of the planet Saturn and relates to patience and emotional control. Therefore, it has a balancing effect on your life.
The **RING** finger connects with the Sun and represents vitality, life energy, and your health. It corresponds to your sense of family and matters of the heart.
The **LITTLE** finger is the indicator for the planet Mercury, which rules your ability to communicate, be creative, appreciate beauty, and achieve inner calm.
The tips of fingers can reveal qualities of different natures.
An oval fingertip can signify an impulsive person who needs motivation. A pointy fingertip is common for an independent, active person, and a square fingertip shows a logical and practical person.

THE CHAKRAS

Within our body, we have seven major nerve and energy centers that are located along the spine. The first is at the base of spine, the seventh at the top of the head. These centers are called Chakras. Their energy is always spinning clockwise within our bodies and influences - and is influenced by – our emotional, spiritual, and physical health. In order to feel balanced and in harmony within ourselves and our environments, it is important that we know about these centers and their functions.

FIRST CHAKRA

Represents: Survival, food, shelter, courage, will, foundation
Location: Base of spine
Gland: Gonads
Color: Red

SECOND CHAKRA

Represents: Sex, creativity, procreation, family, inspiration
Location: Sex organs
Gland: Adrenal
Color: Orange

THIRD CHAKRA

Represents: Ego, emotional center, the intellect, the mind
Location: Solar plexus
Gland: Pancreas
Color: Yellow

FOURTH CHAKRA

Represents: Unconditional true love, devotion, faith, compassion
Location: Heart region
Gland: Thymus
Color: Green or pink

FIFTH CHAKRA

Represents: Voice, truth, communication, higher knowledge
Location: Throat
Gland: Thyroid
Color: Blue

SIXTH CHAKRA

Represents: Third Eye, vision, intuition
Location: Third Eye
Gland: Pineal
Color: Indigo

SEVENTH CHAKRA

Represents: Universal God consciousness, the heavens, unity, humility
Location: Top of the head, crown
Gland: Pituitary
Color: Violet

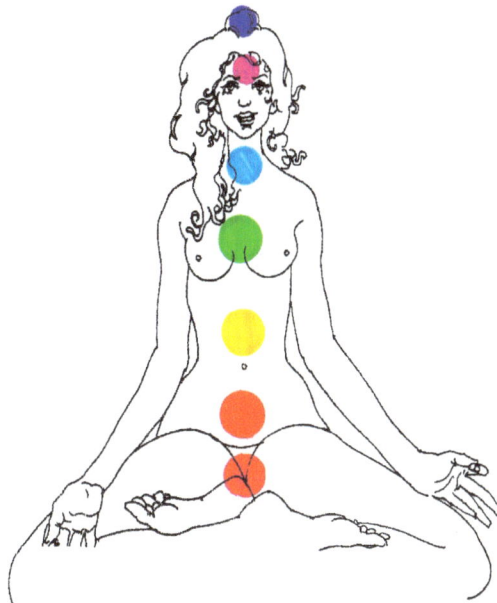

CHAKRAS IN THE BODY

Base Chakra: Foundation
Second Chakra: Sexuality
Third Chakra: Ego
Fourth Chakra: Love
Fifth Chakra: Truth
Sixth Chakra: Intuition
Seventh Chakra: Divine Wisdom

Mudras are a powerful tool for energizing and balancing each Chakra, activating the electric current in our body, and releasing the limitless power from within. Example: When practicing the mudra for divine worship, you can visualize healing Chakra colors surrounding, filling, and energizing your body, starting with the First Chakra and continuing up to your head, the Crown Chakra.

ELECTRIC CURRENTS

Besides the seven Chakras within our body, there are seventy-two thousand electric currents or channels called *Nadis* - pronounced "nah-dees". They run from all different body points, from the tips of the toes to the top of the head. The Nadis also affect your entire system. Keeping these energy currents activated and full of powerful flowing energy is essential to your wellbeing. Each mudra redirects, activates, and empowers the energy flowing through those channels, and stimulates the brain centers, nerves, and organs, with benefits to your entire neuromuscular, physical, and glandular system.

HEALING COLORS

Using the healing power of colors can also enhance your mudra practice. The rainbow colors of the Chakras heal and reenergize corresponding body parts. You can surround yourself with appropriate colors whenever you meditate or visualize the colors as you practice mudras.

For instance, when practicing the mudra for powerful insight, you can visualize yourself surrounded by white or violet light. This will enhance your intuitive capacity. Wearing a certain color will also influence your entire outlook on life.

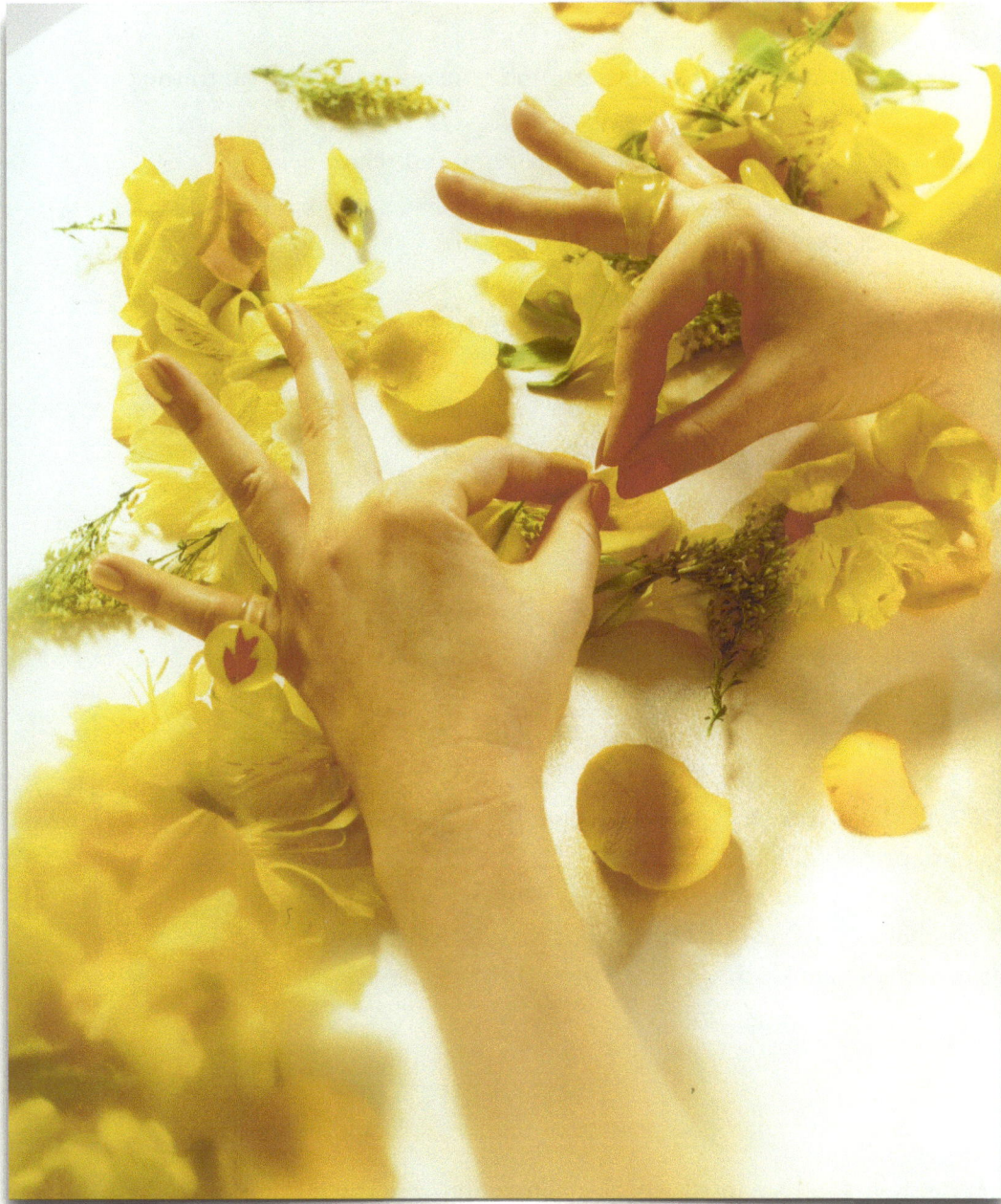

MUDRA OF YIN - FEMININE POWER

Examples:

RED will positively affect your vitality, ground you, and connect you to the earth.

ORANGE will empower your sexuality, creativity, and relationships.

YELLOW makes you feel energized and full of fire.

GREEN is good for the days when you need to heal your heart and feel love.

BLUE has a calming, peaceful effect on your aura or the energy field surrounding your body, and will help you see and speak the truth.

INDIGO will enhance your intuition and sixth sense.

VIOLET is a great centering and calming color that will help you connect with the universal healing powers.

BLACK will help you communicate as the leader.

WHITE will make you feel cleansed and pure, and will help clear you of any negative feelings or depression.

Reflect on the messages your body sends you every morning, and see what color you feel most drawn to and comfortable wearing on different days.

THE AURA

Our aura or energy body is made of electromagnetic energy vibrations that include color, light, sound, heat, and emotions. It surrounds us as a glow that is usually invisible. With practice and concentration, however, you can learn to see auras. The mudra for feeling the energy body is particularly effective in helping you discern auras. When our invisible magnetic force is very vibrant, it signifies good health, personal power, and a healing capacity.

USEFUL MUDRA TIPS

Some mudras may seem at first to be very similar to each other. Yet each is, in practice quite different: every detail in the posture of your hands and fingers is important and significant. When you pay close attention to your practice of mudras, you will feel the difference. As we discussed, every fingertip is connected to a different body center and energy current. Concentrate on the mudra as you practice, and notice the different feeling and effect that each brings to you. You can practice one specific mudra at a time or combine a few in one sitting. Listen to your body.

Example: If you are stressed out and need to concentrate, practice the mudra for preventing stress. After three minutes, go on to the mudra for concentration. As you try different combinations, your body-mind's logic and intuition will guide you. That is the beauty of the mudras – you can practice them anyplace, anytime, in whatever order you desire. This ancient science of the mudra is complex in benefits, yet simple in practice.

Now that you have some background about the power and history of mudras, and some rudiments of meditation practice, you're ready to begin trying some mudras and applying their energy to your life. In the next sections, you will find mudras for your soul, mudras for healing physical conditions, and mudras for easing troublesome states of mind, among others. Every one of these fifty-two traditional mudras can be a spiritual tool for you and help you in your own process of self-discovery and creative problem solving. I hope that they will enable you to find more insight, pleasure, and power on your life journey.

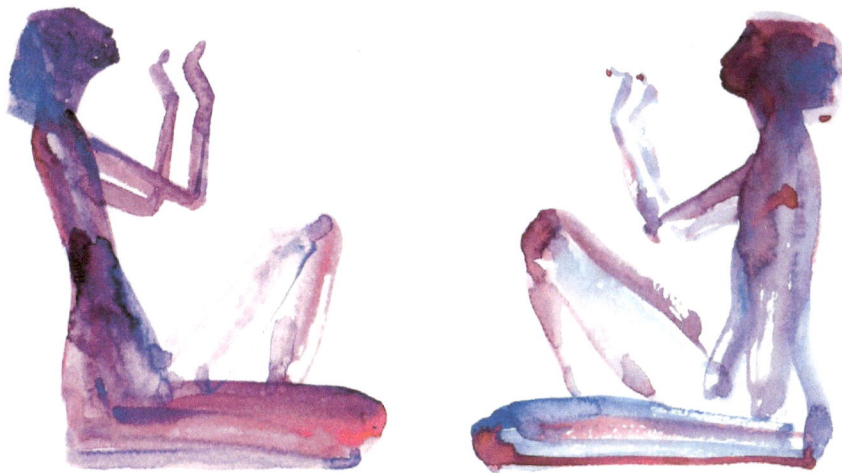

MUDRAS

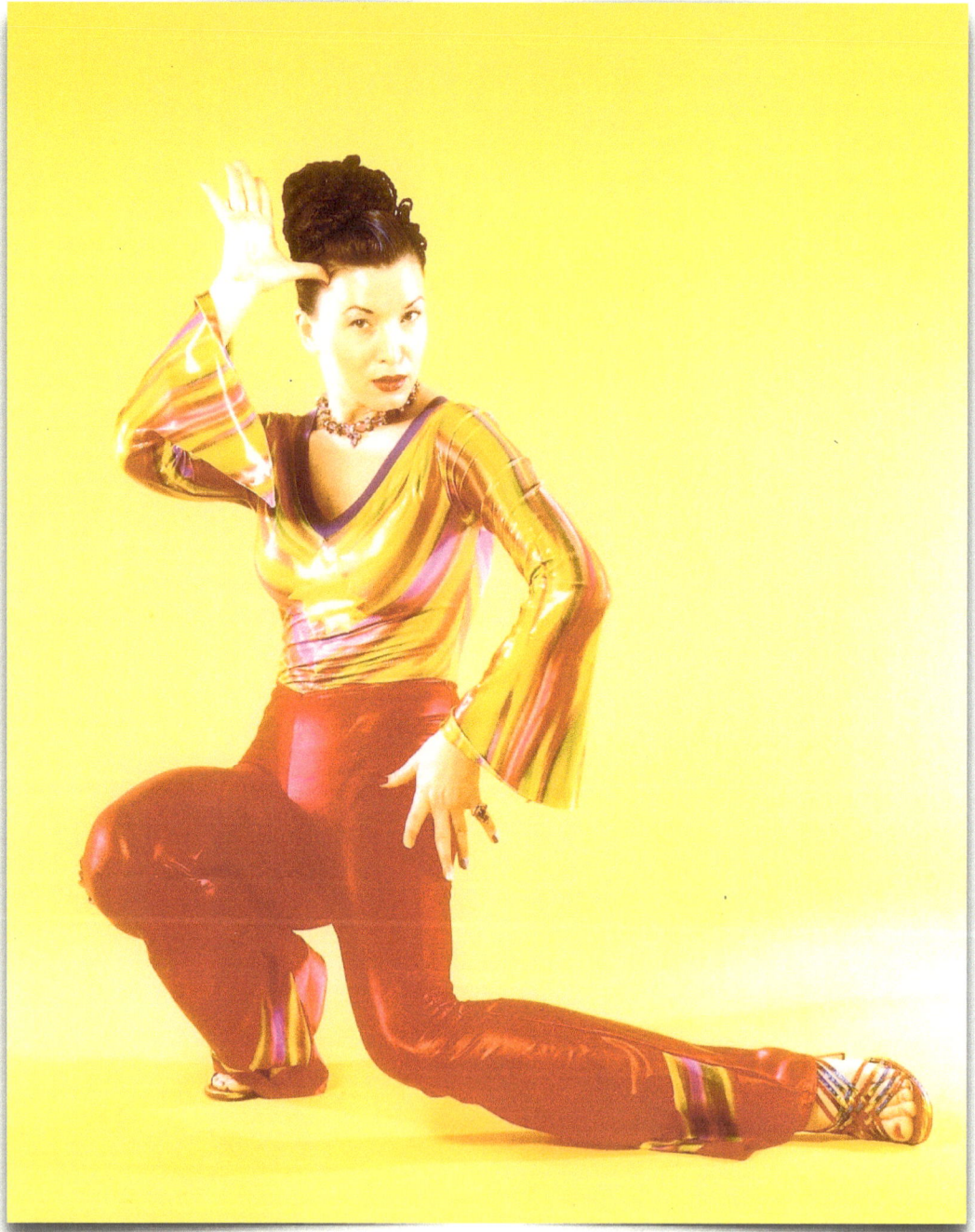

MUDRAS
FOR YOUR MIND

YOUR MIND HAS NO LIMITATIONS...
EXPAND IT.

These twenty-one mudras for the mind are helpful with variety of problems that you have created for yourself – in your mind. A confused state of mind is like a wild horse running. With discipline, you can rein in the energy of your wild thoughts and master your mind. When you teach your mind who is in charge, anything and everything becomes possible. Chase away your self – created ghosts of fear and insecurity and experience the immense power of your mind with these yoga practices.

You have been given a divine gift of free will. What you do with it, you alone decide. We create our own destiny, and with a sharp mind, you can define, correct, and change your destiny for the better.

You can practice one mudra a day or as many as you wish, until your fears and other mental obstacles disappear. As your mind clears, you will see how to use it to help yourself and others. When you act for the good of this planet, you will never be alone.

BEDTIME MUDRA FOR A GOOD MORNING

The way we feel in the morning affects our entire day. Waking up positive and rested, full of energy and inspiration, will help us live a happier, healthier, more fulfilled, and adventurous life.

This mudra must be done at bedtime to give you a positive frame of mind in the morning.
As you practice it, visualize a white ball of light above your head.
You will start the next day protected and surrounded by white light.

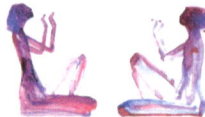

CHAKRA: All Chakras
COLOR: All Colors
MANTRA: HAR HARE WAHE, HAR HARE WAHE
~ God is the Creator of Supreme power and Wisdom ~
Repeat mentally, with six strokes of inhale and one long exhale

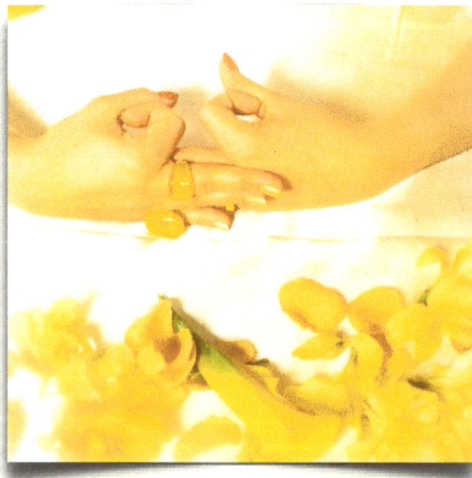

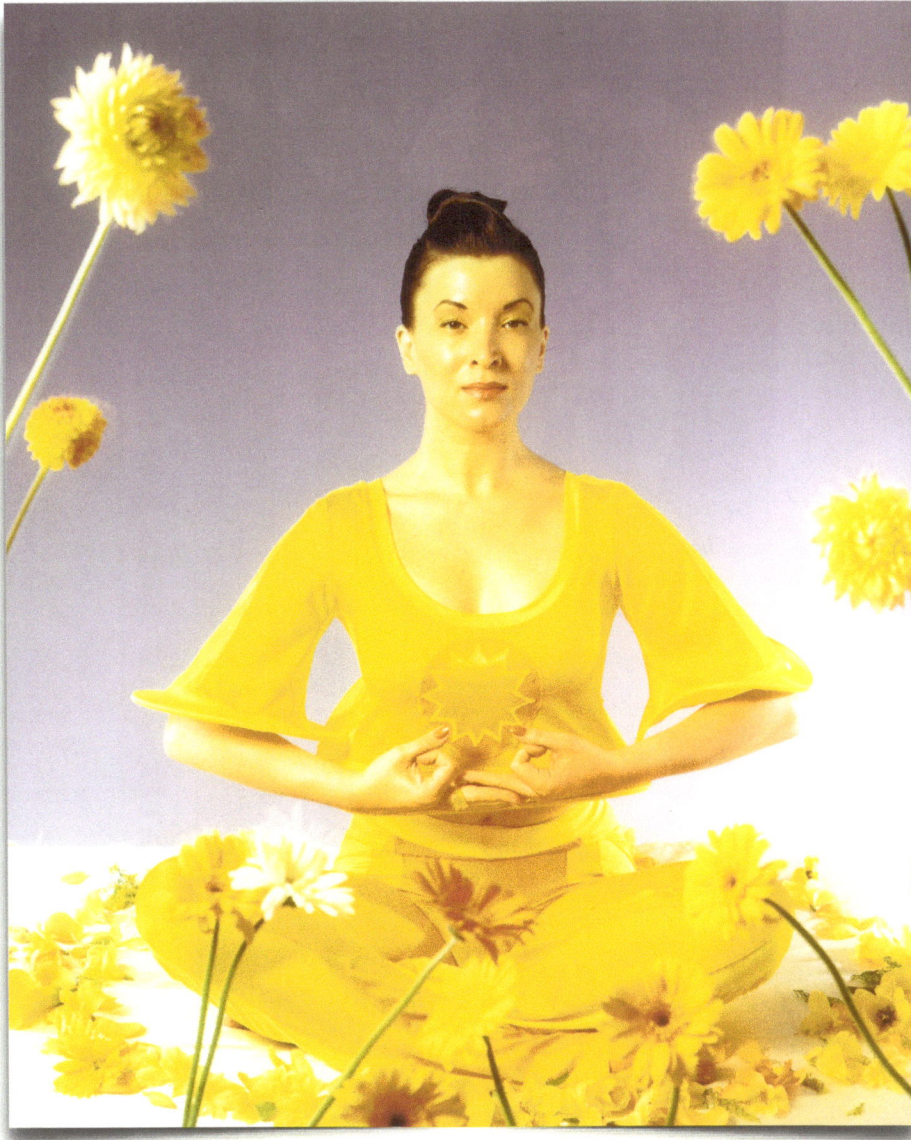

Sit with a straight spine, elbows extended to the sides, hands a few inches in front of the body, just above the navel. Your palms are facing up. Curl your thumbs around the index fingertips and extend the middle, ring, and little fingers so that they touch each other back to back. Keep your palms up, left hand on top of the right.

BREATH: INHALE SIX SHORT BREATHS AS YOU MENTALLY REPEAT THE MANTRA AND EXHALE IN ONE STRONG BREATH. Continue for three minutes and build up your time to eleven minutes.

MUDRA FOR FACING FEAR

Fear prevents us from achieving our goals and dreams. Sometimes the energy you create by being afraid of certain things will actually attract those exact situations into your life. When we give fear too much power over us in our own mind, we may see "our worst fears come true." If this occurs, see it as an opportunity to deal with the fear and conquer it.

The right hand is symbolic of divine protection; the left hand symbolizes your receiving this gift. This mudra will help you diminish all feelings of fear. It is used in many cultures and is very powerful.

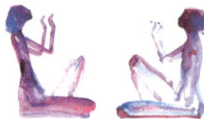

CHAKRA: Solar Plexus - 3
Crown - 7

COLOR: Yellow, violet

MANTRA: NIRBHAO NIRVAIR AKAAL MORT
~ Fearless, Without Enemy, Immortal Personified God ~
Repeat with each breath

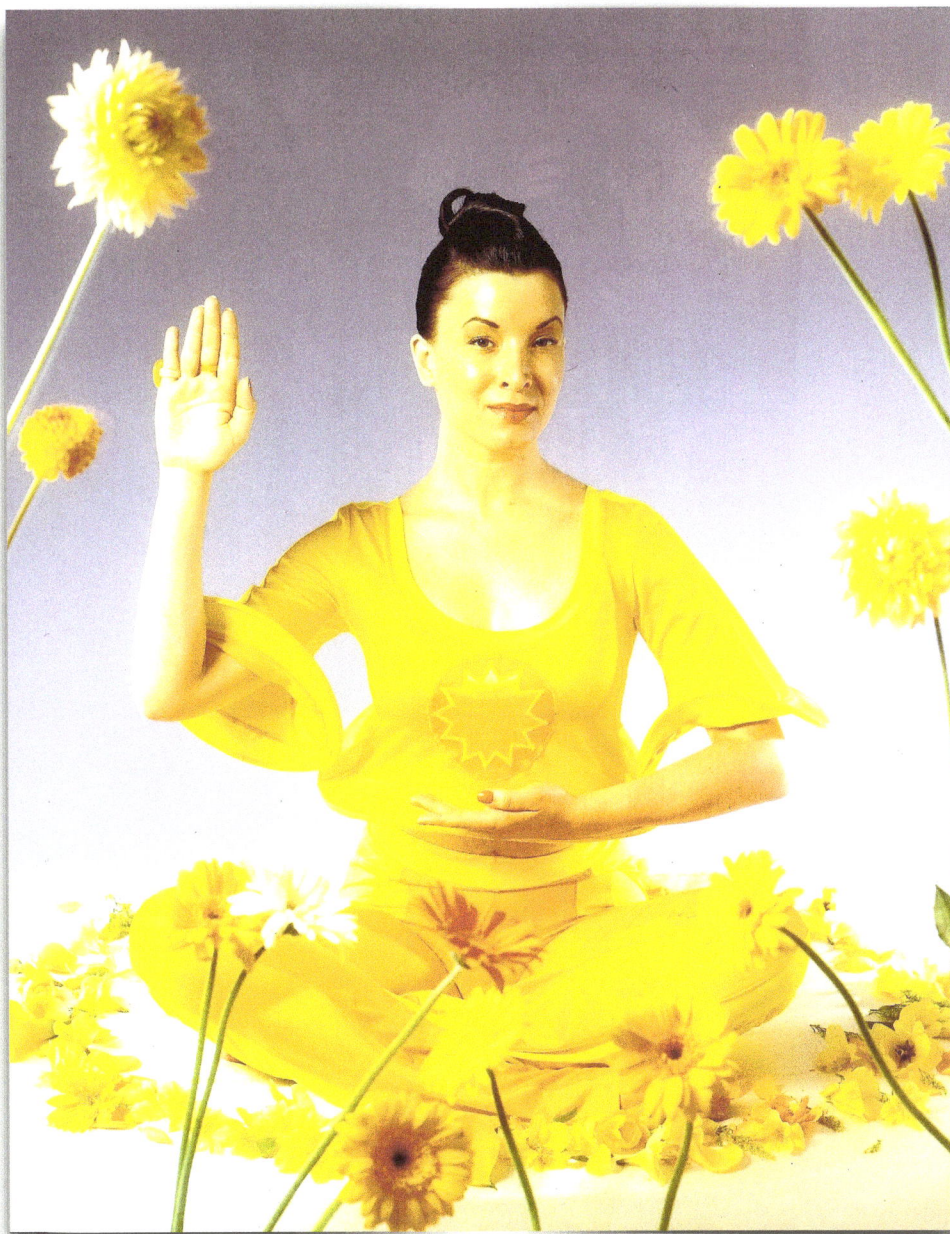

Sit with a straight spine, bend your left arm at the elbow, and hold your hand in front of your navel with the palm up. Lift your right arm and hold your hand in front of your right shoulder with the palm turned outward, fingers and thumb straight up. Concentrate on your Third Eye.

BREATH: LONG, DEEP AND SLOW. See yourself protected, inhale that positive feeling, and exhale the negative fear.

MUDRA FOR RELEASING GUILT

We all carry with us some feelings of guilt. Maybe somewhere in our past we behaved selfishly or angrily. Maybe we feel we don't really deserve to be happy, fortunate, or loved. Negative past experiences can be blocking us from moving forward in our lives with optimism and joy. Forgiving yourself is a necessary step for achieving a fulfilled, healthy, and happy life. The practice of this mudra is the first step to freeing your spirit from the weight of the past.

This mudra stimulates a rejuvenating energy that helps clear your mind and direct it toward new, positive thoughts and possibilities.

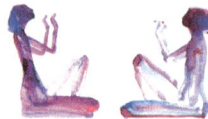

CHAKRA: Solar Plexus - 3

COLOR: Yellow

MANTRA: I AM THINE WAHE GURU
~ I Am Thine, Divine Teacher Within ~
Repeat mentally with each breath

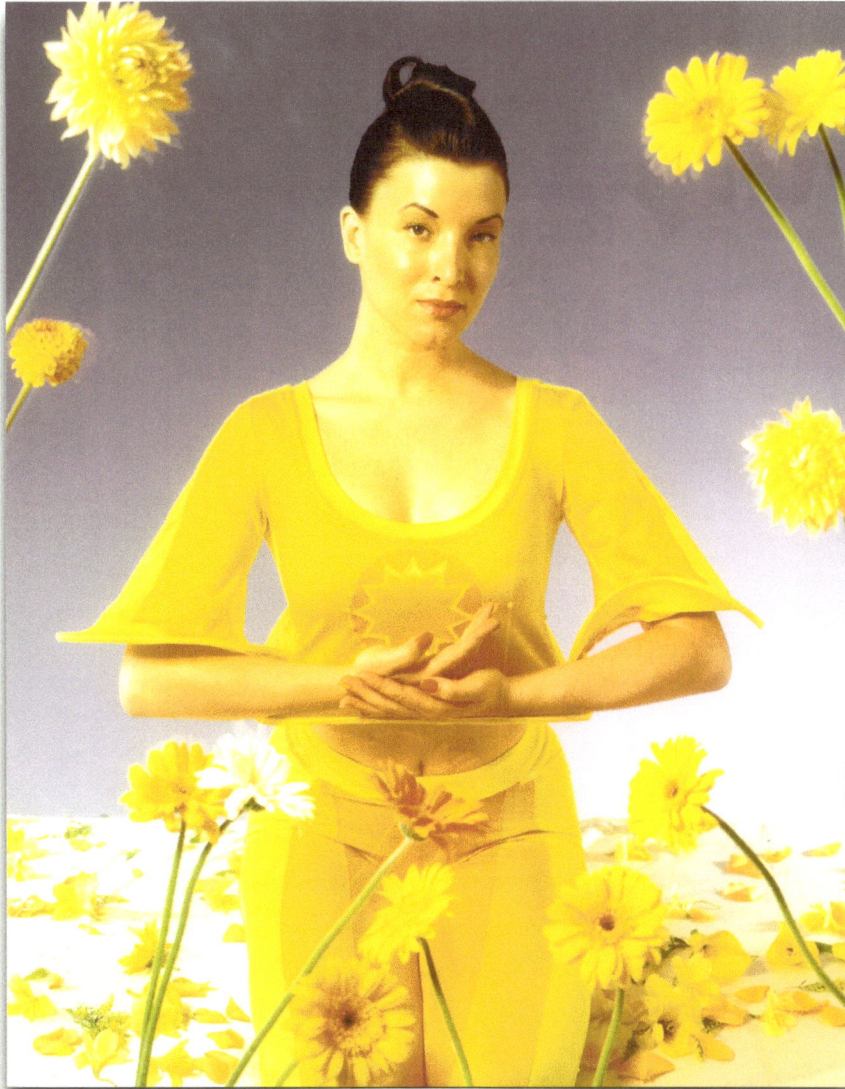

Sit or kneel with a straight back, elbows out to the sides, and bring your palms up to the level between your stomach and heart center. Palms are facing up toward the sky, right hand resting in left. Upper arms are slightly away from the body. Breathe slowly and deeply. Think of the situation that burdens you and release that feeling with each exhalation. Now replace it with a positive affirmation "I forgive myself" and ask the Higher Power to erase any wrongs you may have done.

BREATH: LONG, DEEP AND SLOW. Practice for a few minutes and relax.

MUDRA FOR STRONGER CHARACTER

We all want to have strong, devoted, and loyal friends, life partners, and business associates. To attract people with these qualities into our lives, we must first develop these qualities within ourselves. Passing the moral tests of life – temptation, selfish motivation, and weak character – with which we are faced every day, makes us stronger in our character. Yet if we fail these tests, they will continue to present themselves. The practice of this pose will help you meet these challenges, build a strong character, and attract similar people into your life.

This mudra will change the metabolism of the mind
and develop happiness of the spirit and personal power.

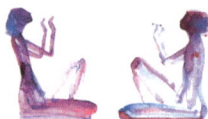

CHAKRA: Solar Plexus - 3
Third Eye - 6

COLOR: Yellow, Indigo

MANTRA: HUMEE HUM BRAHAM
~ Calling on the Infinite Self ~
Repeat mentally with each breath

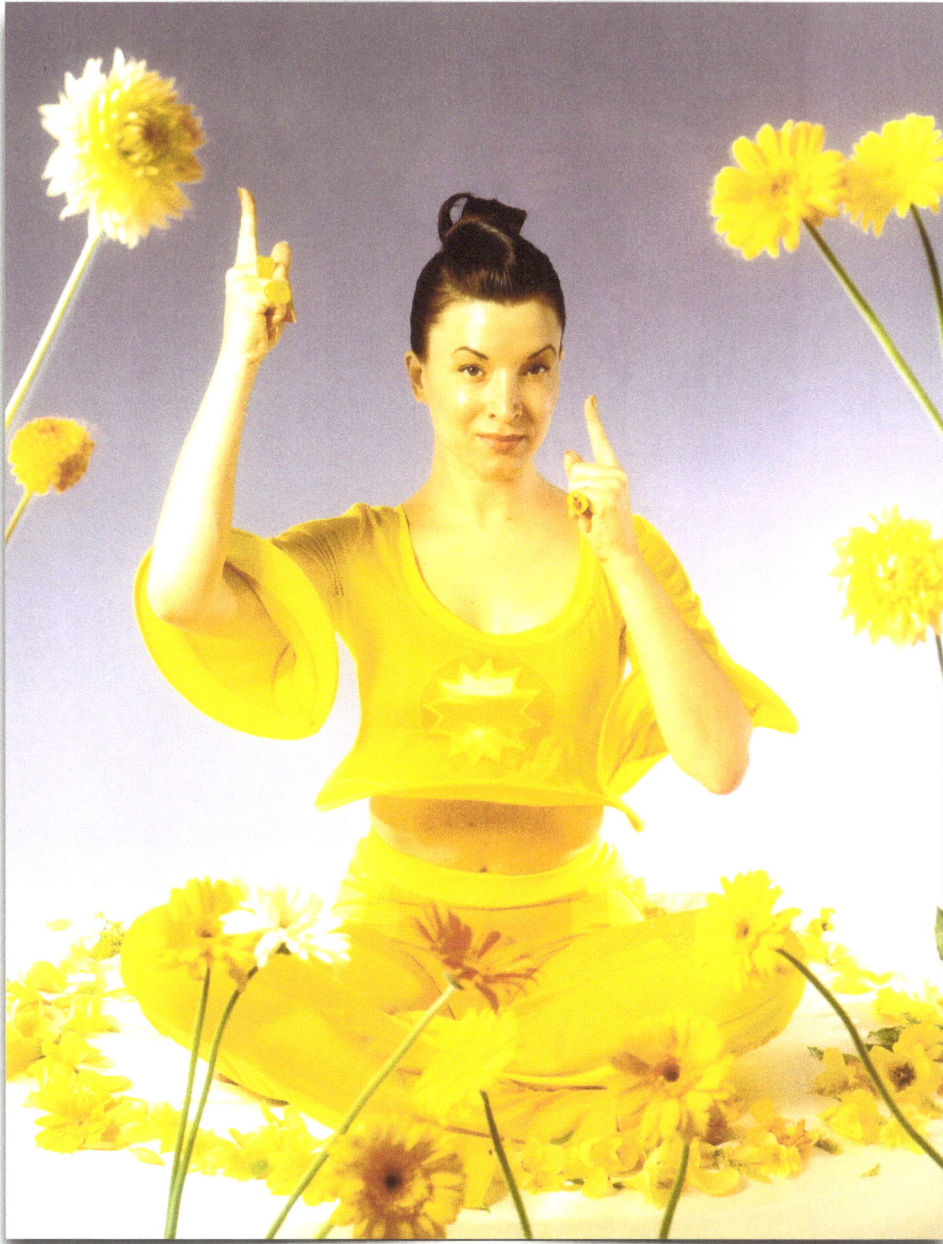

Sit with a straight back and hold your arms at your sides, your hands in relaxed fists. Thumbs are outside, index fingers are straight. Lift your hands up, left hand at the level of your face and right fist slightly above your face. Hands are facing each other. Keep your eyes open and look forward.

BREATH: LONG, DEEP AND SLOW. Repeat for a few minutes and relax.

Mudra for Concentration

The power to concentrate magnifies your capacity to achieve your goals and attract positive experiences and people into your life. Mastering and directing your thoughts is the ultimate goal of concentration and is necessary for your spiritual evolution. You can learn to concentrate with practice.

This mudra helps you become calm while giving you the capacity to focus. It was used by saints and sages when they achieved Samadhi, or the ultimate state of ecstatic meditation.

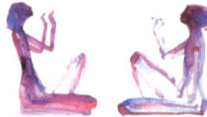

CHAKRA: Solar Plexus – 3
Heart – 4
Third Eye - 6
COLOR: Yellow, Green, Indigo

MANTRA: AKAL AKAL AKAL HARI AKAAL
~ Immortal Creator ~
Repeat mentally with each breath

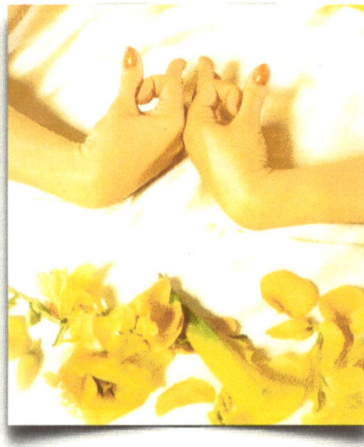

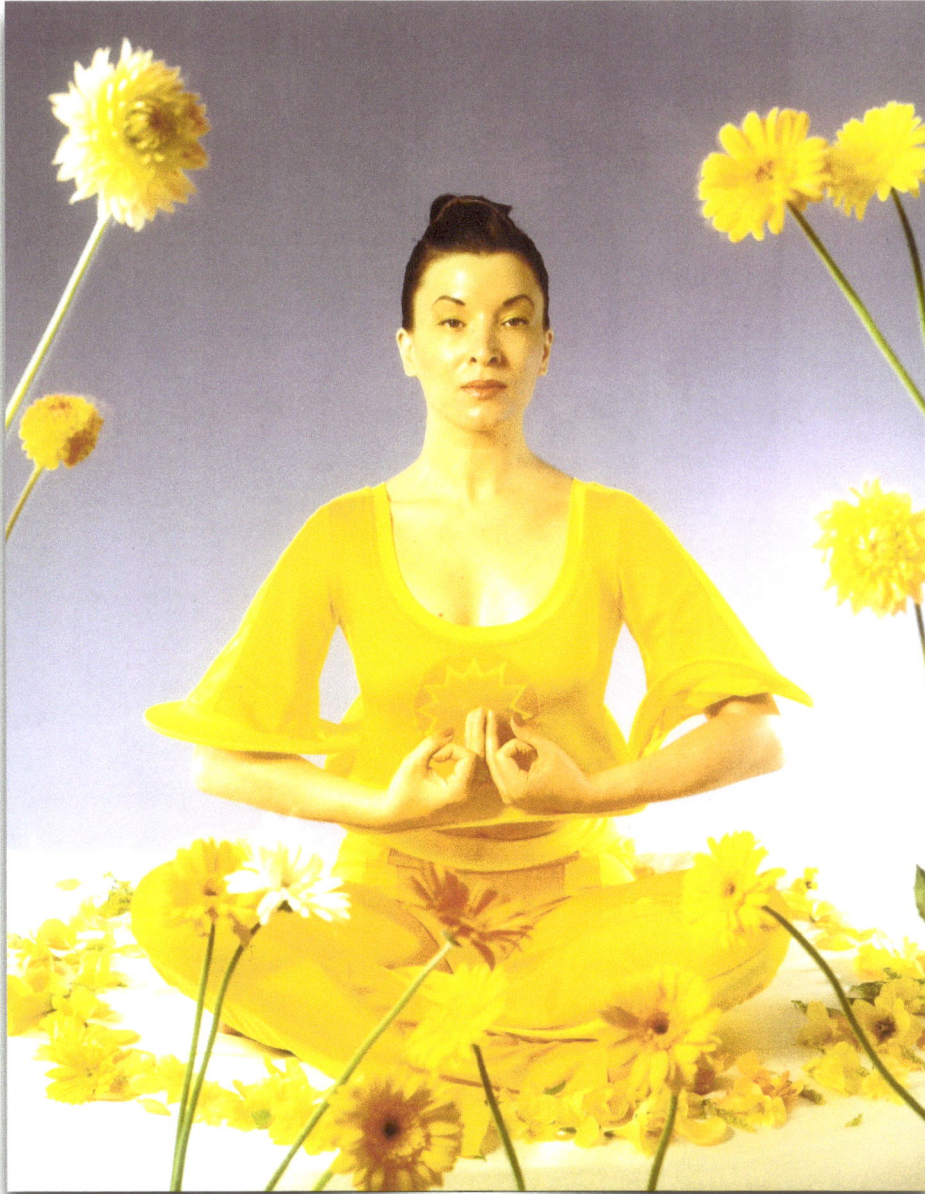

Sit in a comfortable position with a straight spine. Curl each thumb and index finger to create a circle, and keep the rest of the fingers straight, pointing up. Bring your hands in front of you just above your navel so that the up-stretched fingers are touching back to back, pointing toward the sky. Close your eyes and concentrate on your Third Eye area.

BREATH: LONG, DEEP AND SLOW. Still your mind and concentrate on a positive affirmation such as :" I AM the eternal light of the world…"

MUDRA FOR OVERCOMING ANXIETY

Anxiety is a frequent reaction to the demands and stress of our daily lives. You can control your anxiety with regular daily practice of this mudra. You can also defuse a sudden anxiety attack by immediately practicing this mudra for a few minutes. You will instantly feel the difference and become more calm and centered.

This mudra creates its calming effect on your nerves by making
a vortex of energy with each hand, which
acts like a vent for your anxious energy.

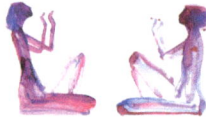

CHAKRA: Solar Plexus – 3
Heart - 4
COLOR: Yellow, Green
MANTRA: HARKANAM SAT NAM
~ God's Name Is Truth ~
Repeat mentally with each breath

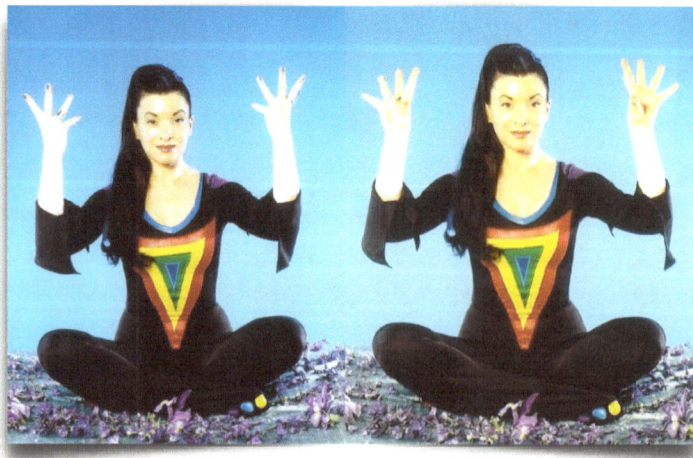

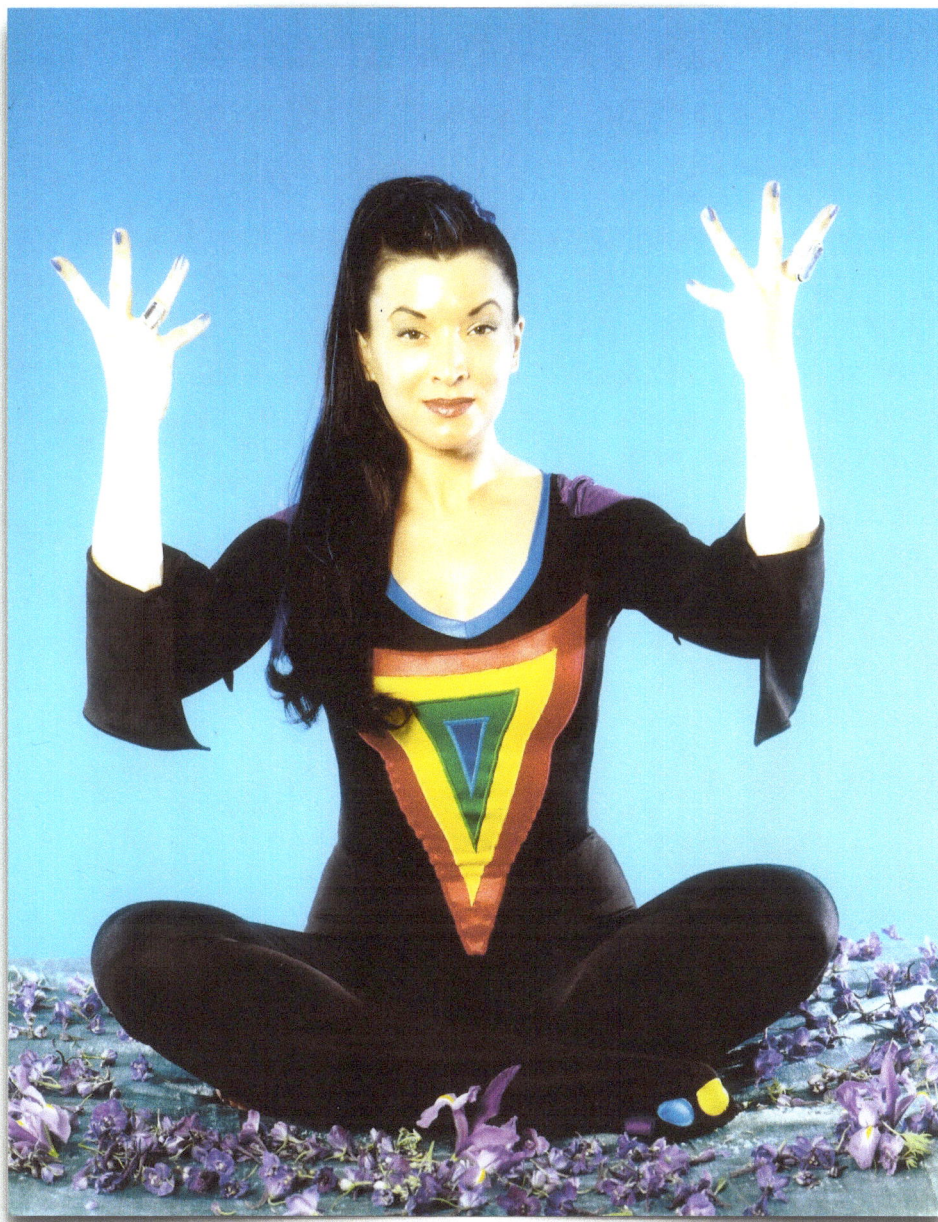

Sit with a straight spine. Bend your elbows and raise your arms so your upper arms are parallel to the ground and extended out to the sides. Your hands should be held at ear level, with fingers spread and pointing toward the sky. Rotate your hands back and forth, pivoting at the wrists. Continue for a few minutes and relax.

BREATH: LONG, DEEP AND SLOW.

Mudra for Transcending Anger and Preventing Headache

We all have the right to get upset at times, but harboring negative emotions is not productive or healthy. To help you transcend angry feelings and figure out how to express them appropriately, practice this mudra. Its immediate and powerful effect will help you channel your anger into a positive outcome or decision. This mudra is also effective for preventing and curing headaches if you have a tendency to get them frequently.

This mudra works by creating an emotional equilibrium.
The pressure points stimulated with your thumbs release anger
and have an immediate calming effect.

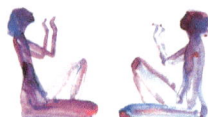

CHAKRA: All Chakras

COLOR: All Colors

MANTRA: GOD AND I, I AND GOD ARE ONE
Repeat mentally with each breath.

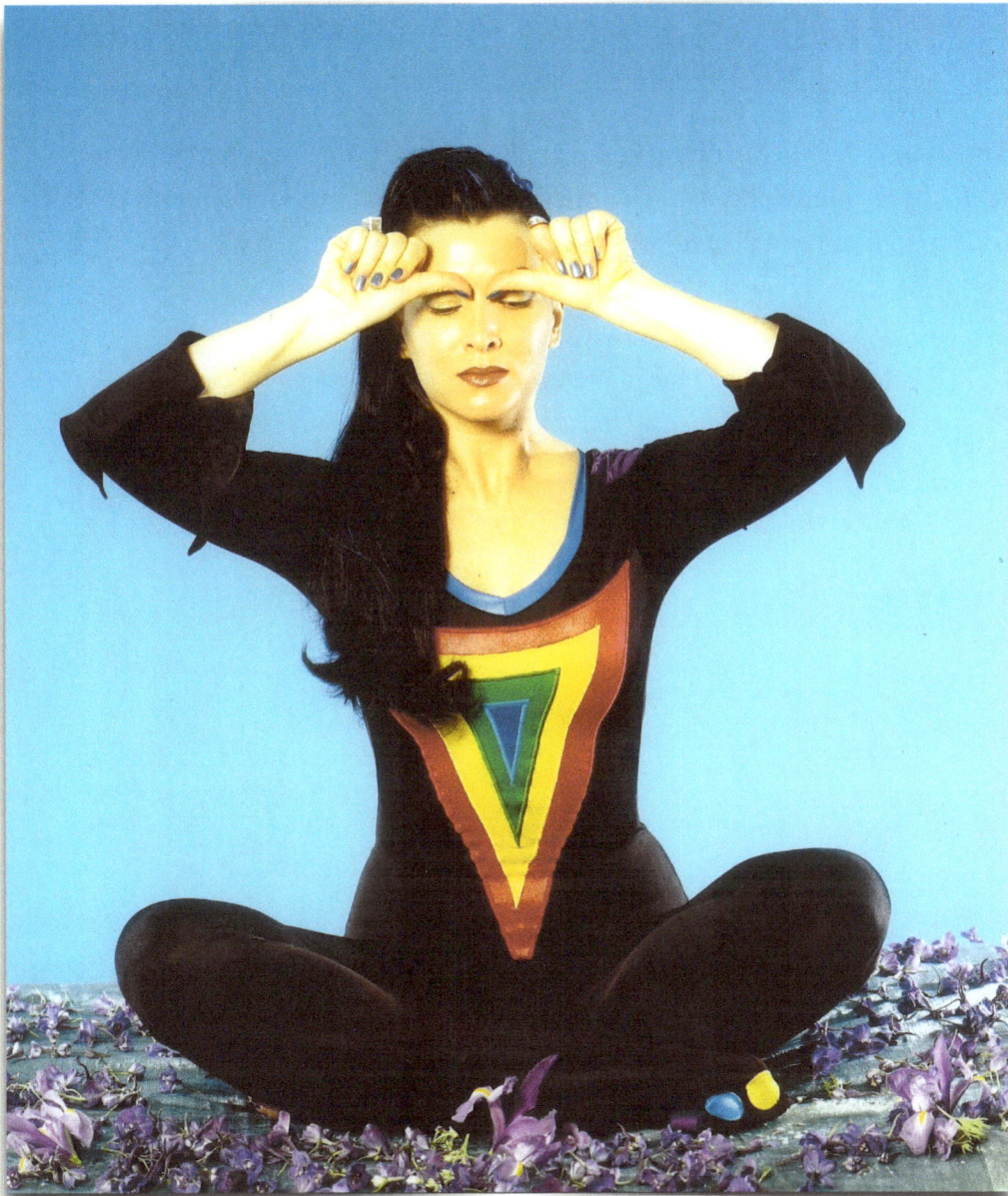

Sit in a comfortable position with a straight spine. Lift your hands to the level of your forehead. Make fists with the palms facing outward and keep the thumbs stretched pointing toward each other. Press the spot on your brow between your eyes and nose and focus your eyes at the tip of your nose.

BREATH: LONG, DEEP AND SLOW.

Continue for three minutes and relax.

MUDRA FOR SHARP MIND

This mudra will help you make up your mind, particularly when you are faced with life-changing decisions. Regular practice of this mudra three times a day for three minutes will give you results in one week.

This mudra neutralizes the central part of the brain and gives you a sharp mind. The moving fingers are stimulating and massaging the meridian that affects your patience, emotional control, solar plexus, nerves, and vitality.

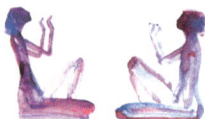

CHAKRA: Throat - 5
Third Eye - 6

COLOR: Blue, Indigo

MANTRA: HARA HARE HARI
~ The Creator in Action ~
Repeat mentally with each breath

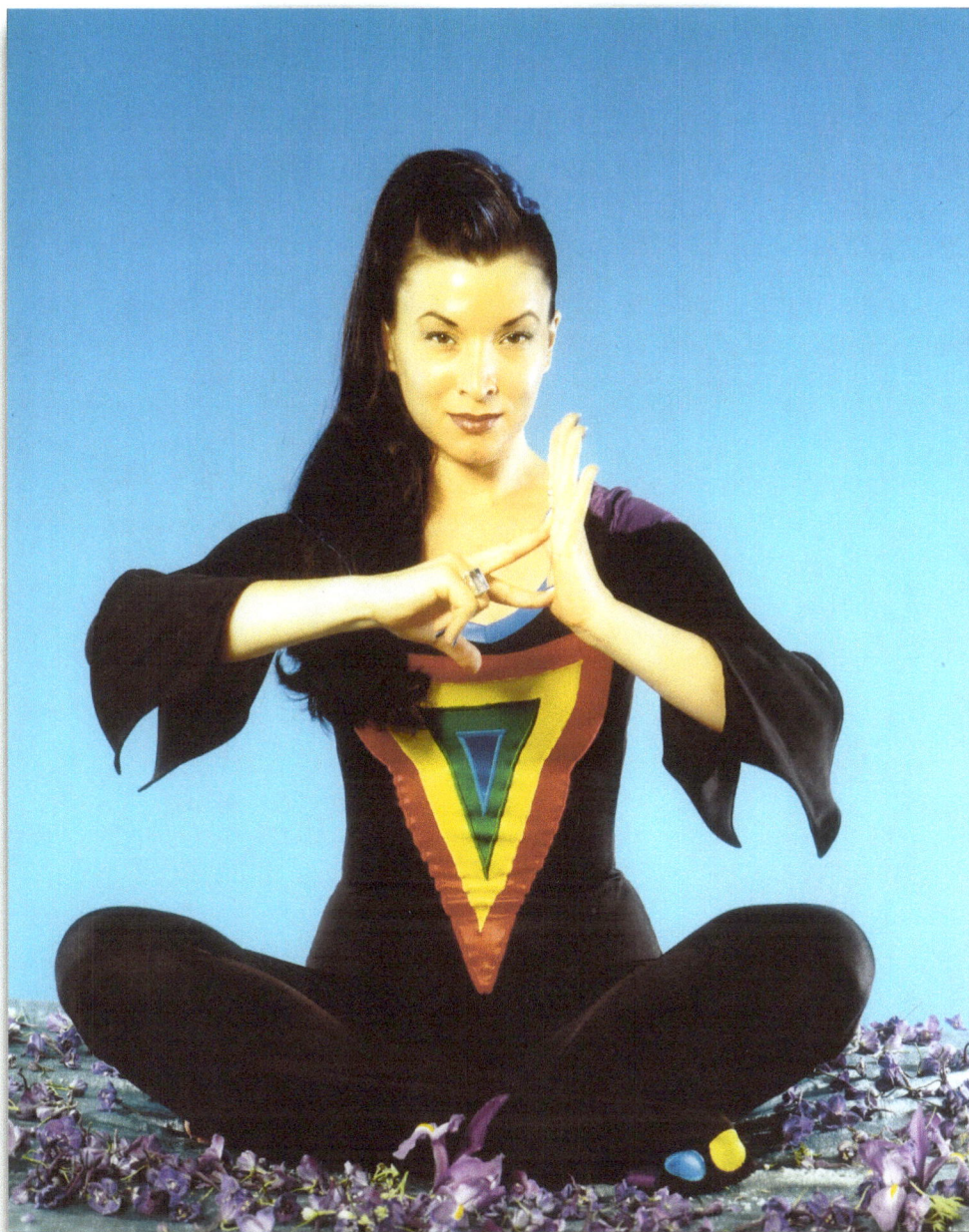

Sit with a straight back. Hold the left hand up as though to clap, then, with the index and middle fingers of the right hand, slowly and with strong pressure walk up the center of the left palm to the very tips of the middle and ring fingers. The left fingers should give in under pressure. Walk up and down a few times while concentrating on the movement of your fingers.

BREATH: LONG, DEEP AND SLOW.

MUDRA FOR PATIENCE

Patience is a virtue that everyone can develop. It is an important component of a happier, healthier life. Remember: In anything you do, after you have done your very best, relax and practice patience. Tell yourself that everything is happening at the right time, even when it seems to make no sense, and you will help make it so.

This mudra will help you transform your frustration and allow you to become more patient and tolerant. Your hands activate electric currents that channel healing energy to your nerves, thus calming you and helping you achieve patience.

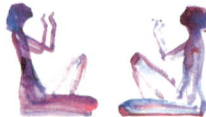

CHAKRA: Third Eye - 6
Crown - 7

COLOR: Indigo, Violet

MANTRA: EK ONG KAR SAT GURU PRASAAD
~ One Creator, Illuminated by God's Grace ~
Repeat mentally with each breath

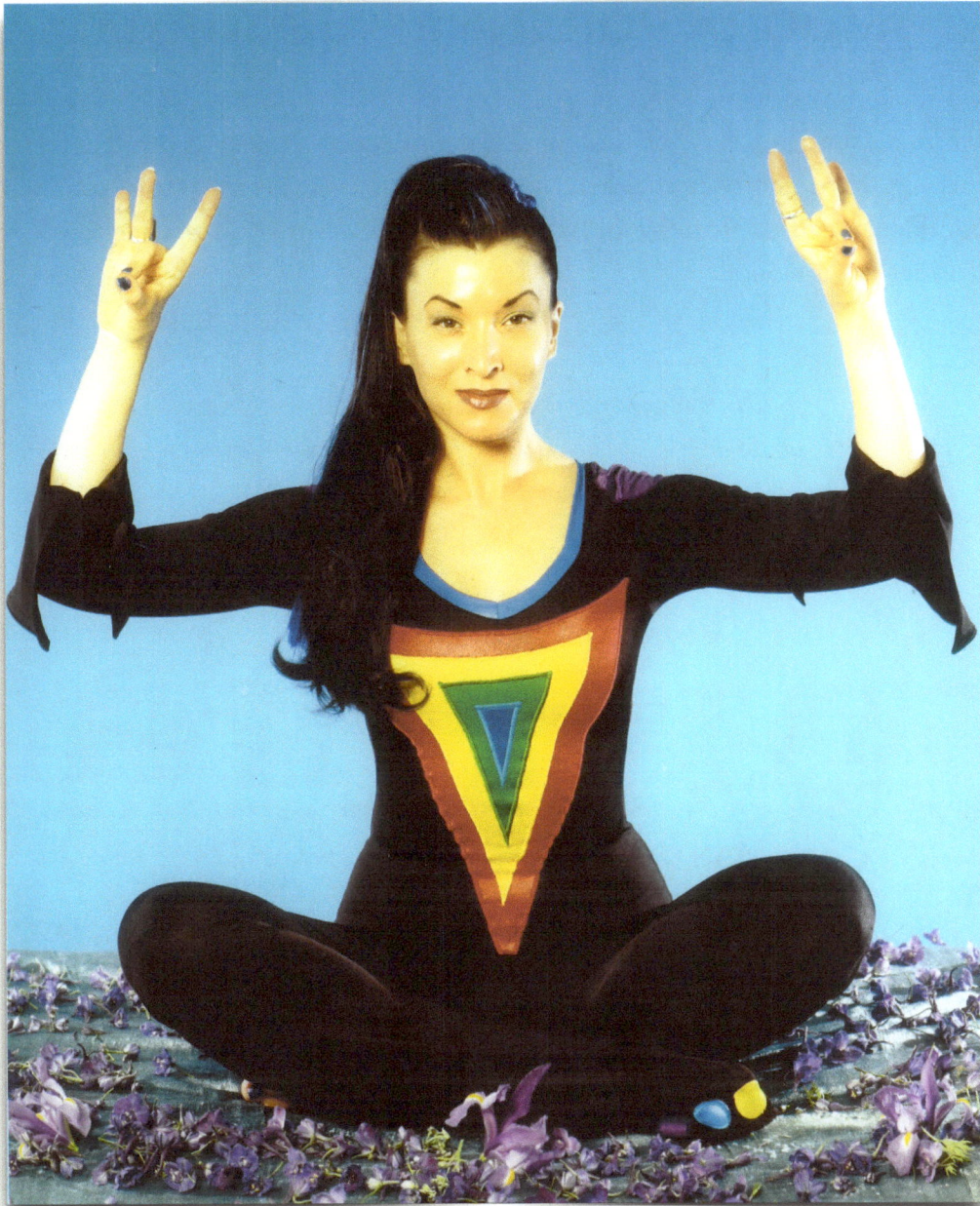

Sit with straight back. Make circles with the tips of your thumbs and middle fingers, keeping the other fingers straight. Upper arms are parallel to the floor, elbows out to the sides. Your hands are at the level of your ears, fingers pointing toward the sky, palms facing front.

BREATH: LONG, DEEP AND SLOW. Repeat for a few minutes and observe yourself becoming calmer and more patient with each breath.

MUDRA FOR INNER SECURITY

Every day brings a new test of our self-confidence. Whenever you feel lost in this big world and overwhelmed by doubts, this mudra will restore your self-confidence and reinforce your sense of inner security. You must remember: You are never alone.

*This mudra works in a positive and empowering way
on the area of the brain that affects your sense of security.*

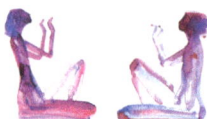

CHAKRA: Solar Plexus - 3
Heart - 4
COLOR: Yellow, green
MANTRA: AD SHAKTI AD SHAKTI
~ I Bow to Creator's Power ~
Repeat mentally with each breath

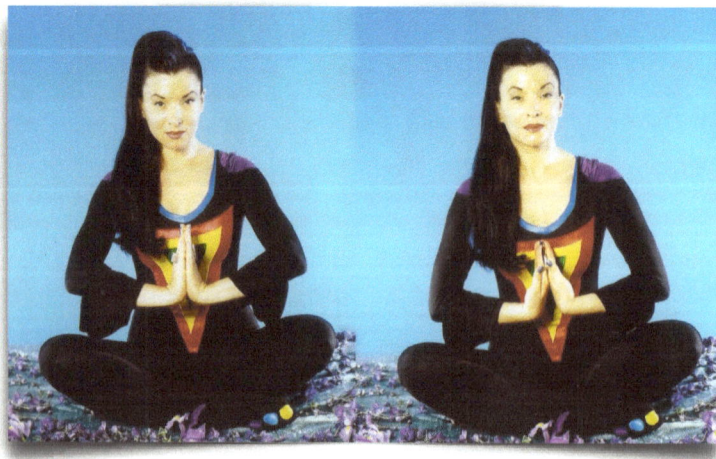

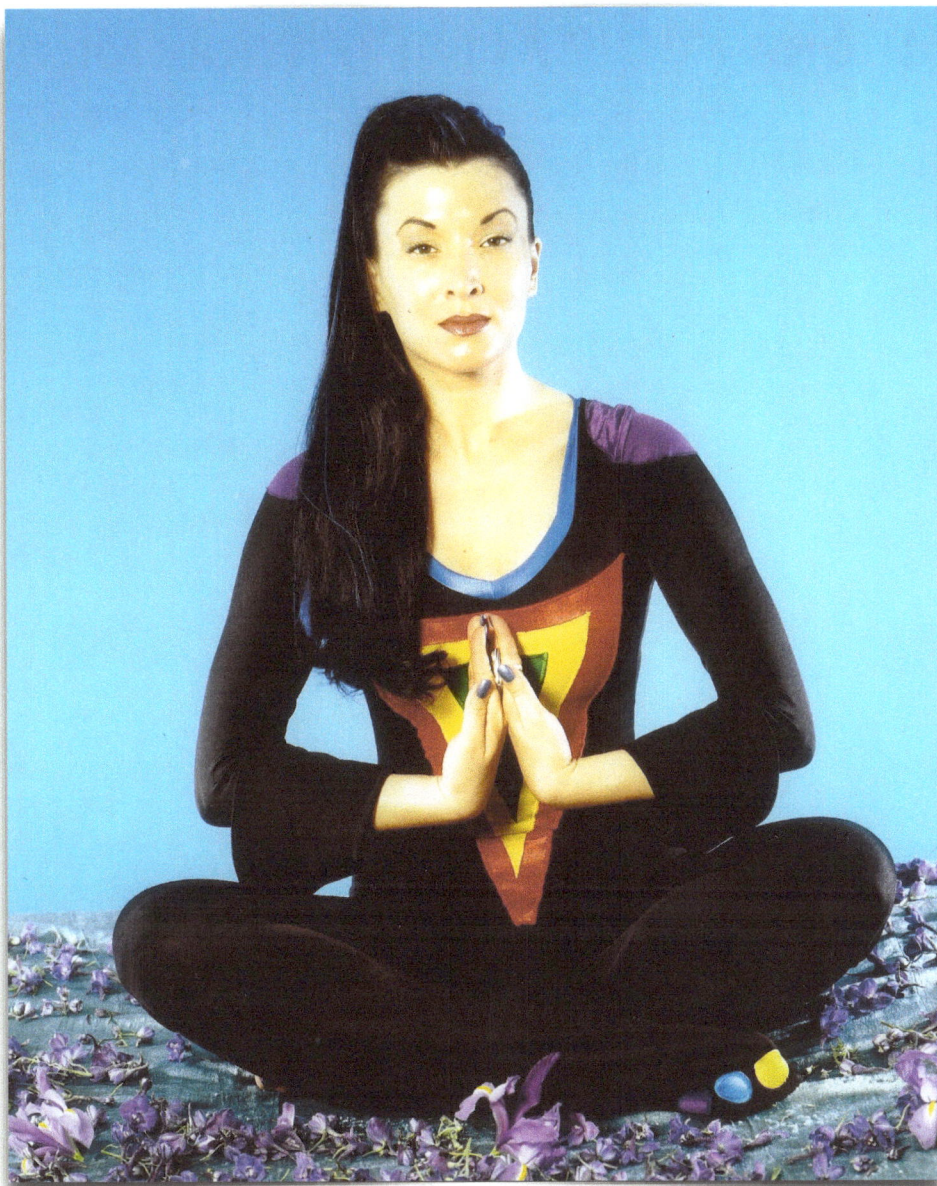

Sit with a straight spine and place you hands in a reversed prayer pose with hands touching back to back. Hold your hands in front of your heart. Imagine the energy moving from the bottom of your spine upward toward the top of your head. Hold the pose for a beat, then reverse the hands into a prayer pose with palms pressed together, thumbs against the chest. Hold for a beat and repeat until you feel calm and secure.

BREATH: LONG, DEEP, AND SLOW

MUDRA FOR CALMING YOUR MIND

A calm mind will give you the ability to center and focus your thoughts and so give you a tremendous capacity for success. The calmer your mind, the more you notice the unrest of others, and faster you can achieve your goals.

This mudra stimulates your brain in a way that calms
your mental activity and helps you control your focus.

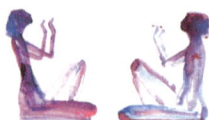

CHAKRA: Solar Plexus - 3
Heart – 4
Third Eye- 6

COLOR: Yellow, Green, Indigo

MANTRA: AKAL HARE HARI AKAL
~ God Is Immortal in His Creation ~
Repeat mentally with each breath

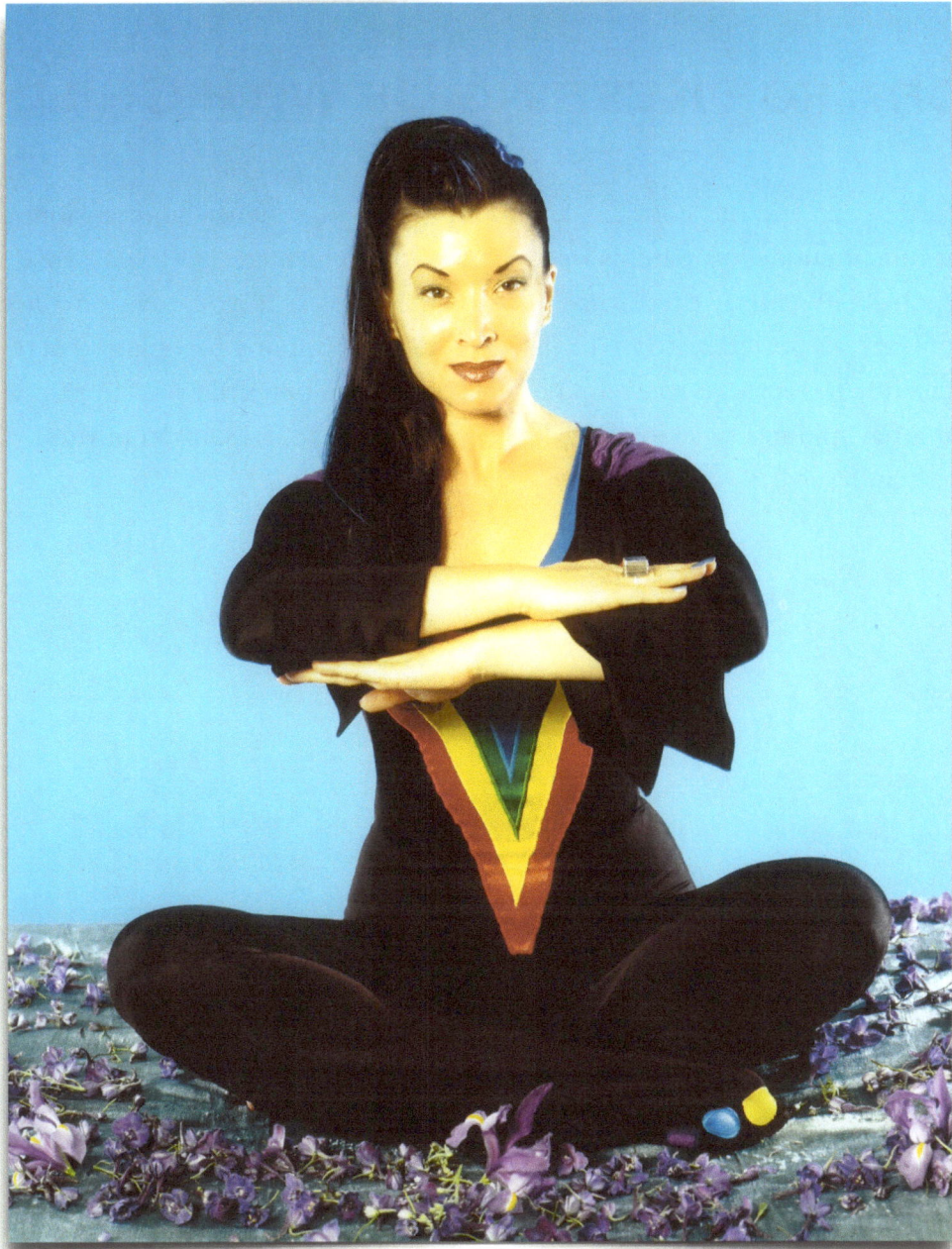

Sit with a straight back and cross your arms in front of your chest, elbows bent at a ninety-degree angle. Arms are parallel to the ground. Place the right palm on top of the left arm and the top of the left hand under the right arm. Fingers are together and straight. Hold this mudra and concentrate for a few minutes, then relax. **BREATH:** LONG, DEEP AND SLOW.

MUDRA FOR KEEPING UP WITH CHILDREN

Children demand our constant attention, guidance, patience, and wisdom. It's not uncommon for parents to become overwhelmed by their sense of responsibility and to need some time to themselves. If you have only a few moments to get away from it all, it is most important to utilize that time efficiently to recharge yourself. This mudra can be practiced on the run, with just a few minutes to spare. It will do wonders for your ability to nurture your children.

This mudra will help you prepare to meet the needs
of parenting on all levels.

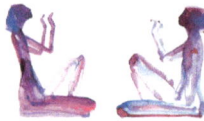

CHAKRA: All Chakras

COLOR: All Colors

MANTRA:
AAD SUCH, JUGAAD SUCH
HAI BHEE SUCH, NANAK HOSEE BHEE SUCH
~ True in the Beginning, True in All Ages,
True at Present, True It Shall Ever Be ~
Repeat mentally with each breath

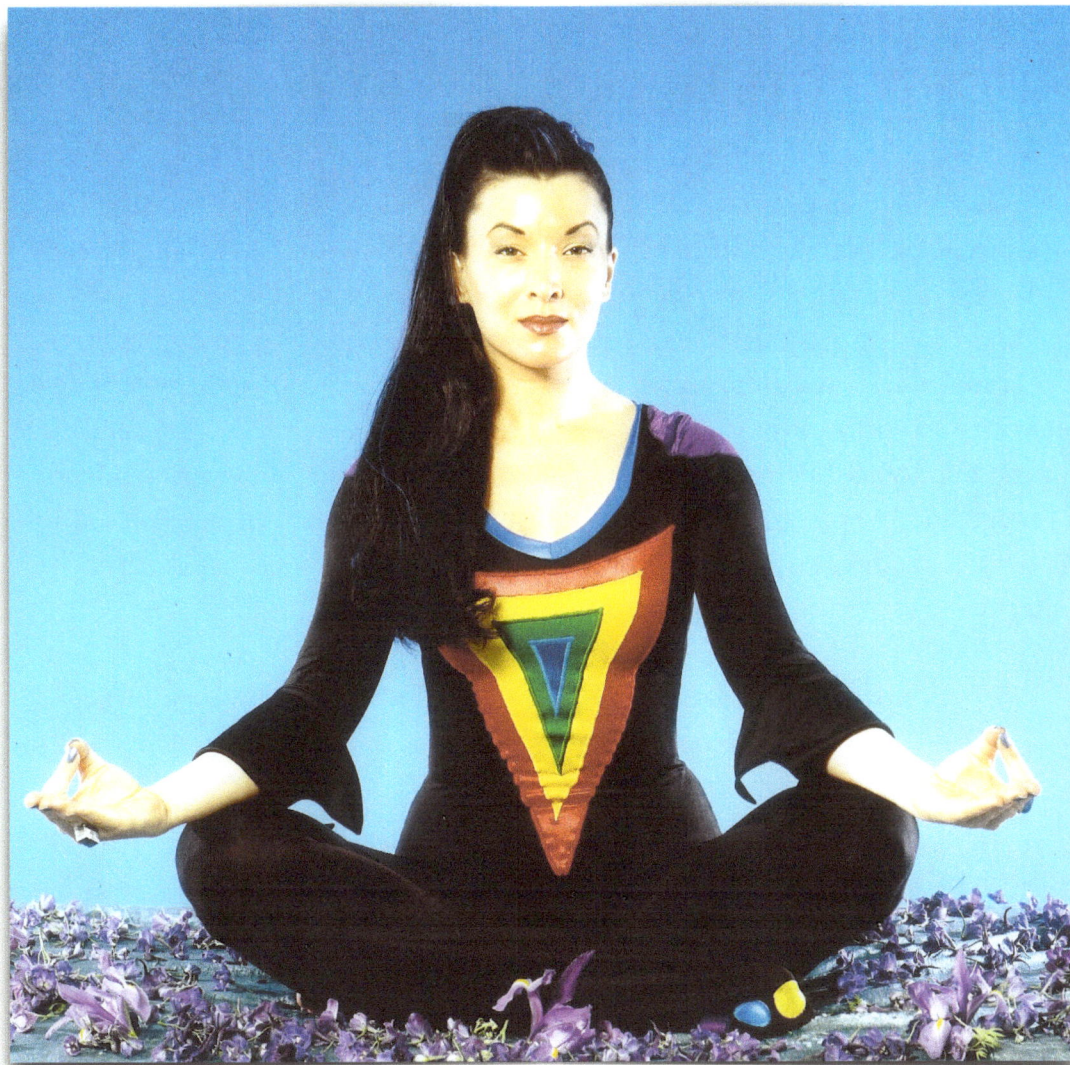

Sit with a straight spine. Make circles with the tips of the thumbs and index fingers. The other fingers are slightly relaxed but extended outward, while the hands rest on the knees. Concentrate on the Crown Chakra.

BREATH: LONG, DEEP AND SLOW.

Continue for three minutes and relax.

MUDRA FOR TAKING AWAY HARDSHIPS

Challenges are an unavoidable part of life. Instead of seeing them negatively as struggles, ask yourself to form the intention to see them as perfectly planned opportunities for your spiritual growth. If you feel that you have had a few cases of "bad luck" and that you have become set in a pattern of pessimism and hardship, you may be creating the kind of energy that will attract such situations on an even greater scale. With this mudra, you can keep your mind and brain patterns on a positive frequency and attract positive energy and people into your life. Hardship and suffering can be replaced by power and strength, but it is your decision what your mindset is going to be. Regular practice will change your life.

This mudra works on the central channel of energy in your body and creates a vibration that takes away hardship and opens the way for positive energy.

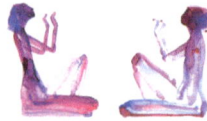

CHAKRA: Third Eye – 6
Crown - 7
COLOR: Indigo, Violet
MANTRA: HAR HARE GOBINDAY, HAR HARE MUKUNDAY
~ He Is My Sustainer, He Is My Liberator ~
Repeat mentally with each breath

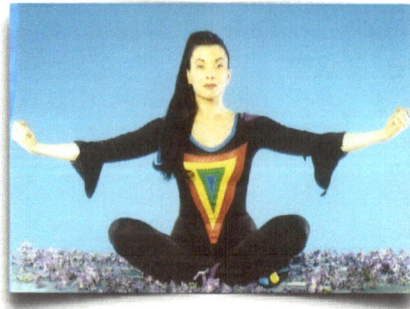

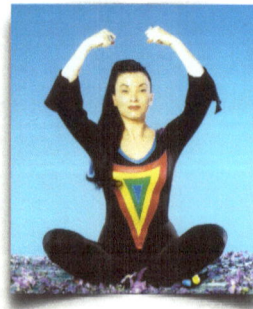

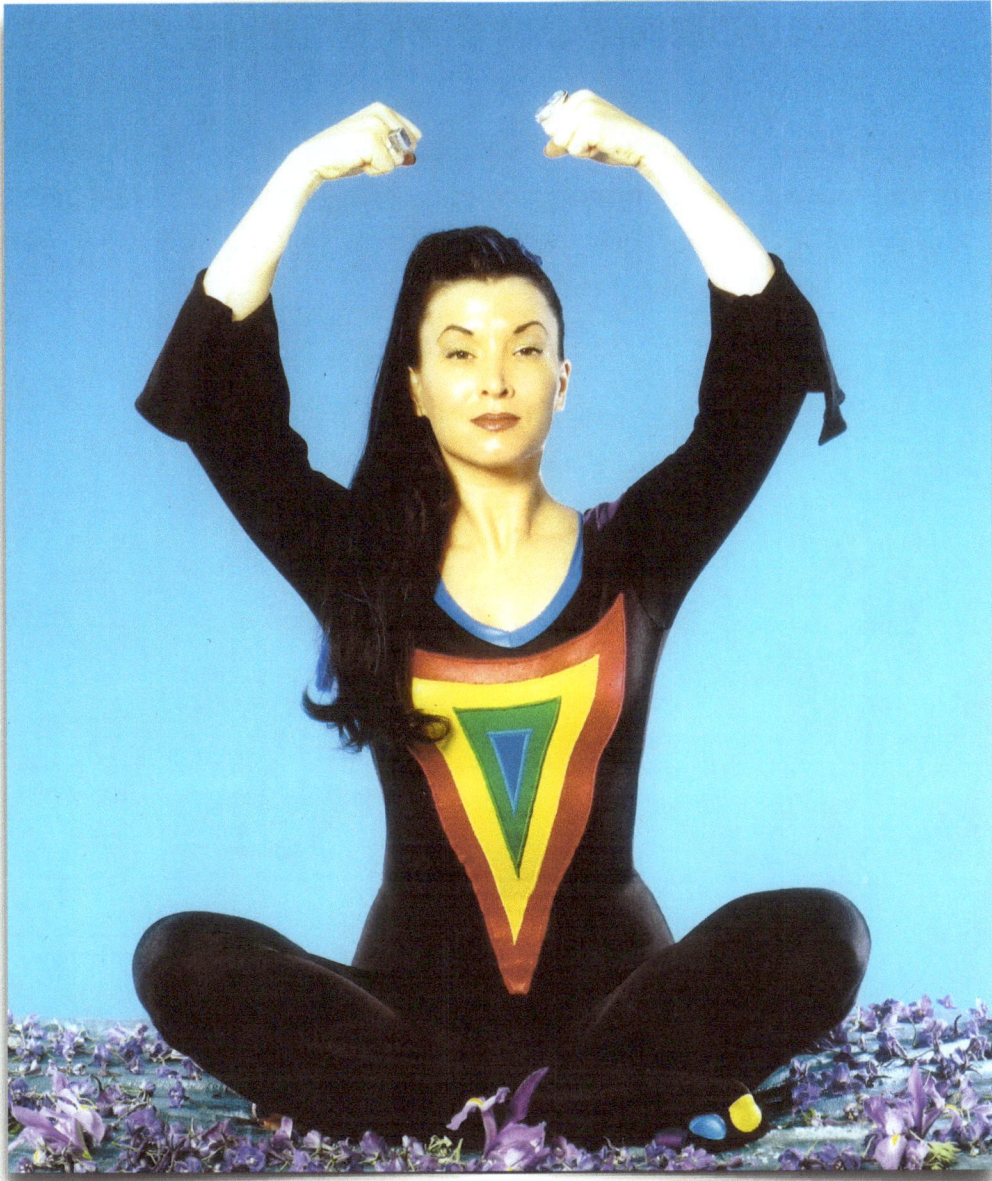

Sit with a straight back and make fists with both hands, thumbs outside. Begin swinging the arms backward in big circles, like a pendulum. First they go forward and up, and then they go back and down.

BREATH: LONG, DEEP AND SLOW.

Continue for a few minutes. Relax and sit still.

MUDRA FOR EFFICIENCY

How many times have you been in a difficult situation and just did not feel sharp and focused enough to deal with it? Even a few minutes of doing this mudra before a meeting, exam, or confrontation will empower you to deal with the situation in the best possible way.

This mudra affects all the electric currents in your body,
brings the entire nervous and glandular system into
balance, and gives razor-sharp efficiency.

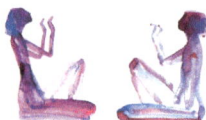

CHAKRA: Heart - 4
Third Eye - 6

COLOR: Green, Indigo

MANTRA: ATMA PARMATMA GURU HARI
~ Soul, Supreme Soul, the Teacher in His Supreme Power and Wisdom ~
Repeat mentally with each breath

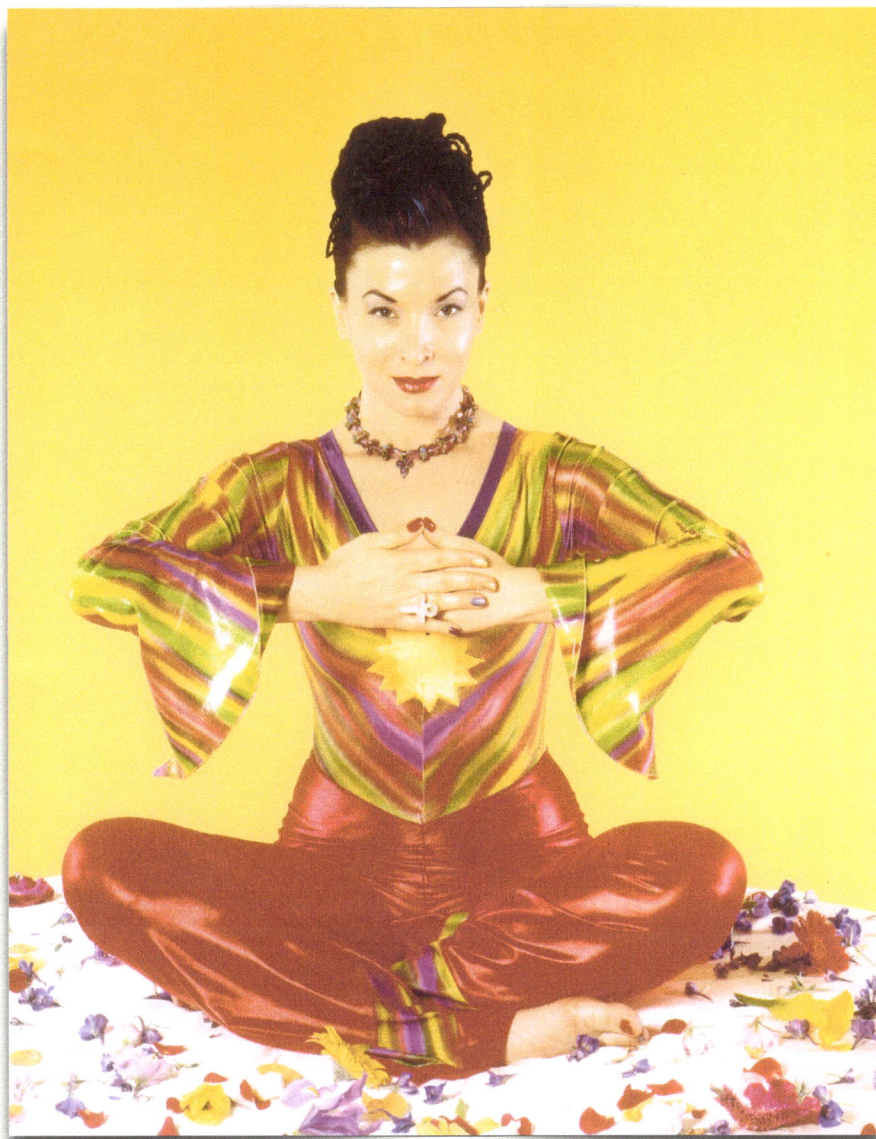

Sit with a straight spine. Bend your elbows, and raise your hands, palms facing your chest, so they overlap and touch at the level of your heart a few inches away from the body. The fingers of both hands are extended, palms facing the body. The palm of the right hand is placed over the back of the left. Press the thumb tips together and hold the hands and forearms parallel to the ground.
BREATH: INHALE DEEPLY AND SLOWLY, HOLD THE BREATH FOR TEN SECONDS, AND EXHALE FOR TEN SECONDS. Wait ten seconds before inhaling again. Continue for a few minutes and relax.

MUDRA FOR TRANQUILIZING THE MIND

A calm ocean or sea…that's how our minds should be. It may take as long as a week of daily practice of this mudra to help you lead a calmer and more peaceful life. But it will work.

This ancient mudra was given by Buddha to his disciples to please and tranquilize their minds. It short-circuits worried, obsessive energy and replaces it with a calming, helpful vibration.

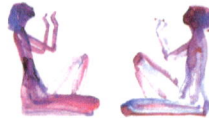

CHAKRA: Solar Plexus – 3
Heart – 4
Throat – 5
Third Eye - 6
COLOR: Yellow, Green, Blue, Indigo
MANTRA: MAN HAR TAN HAR GURU HAR
~Mind with God, Soul with God,
the Divine Guide and His Supreme Wisdom ~
Repeat mentally with each breath.

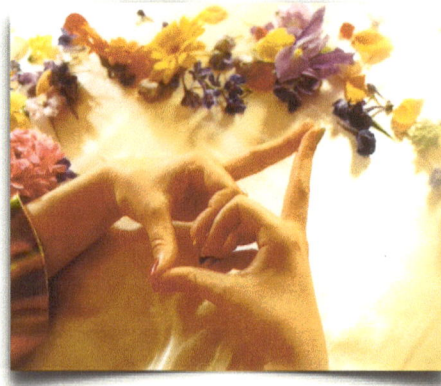

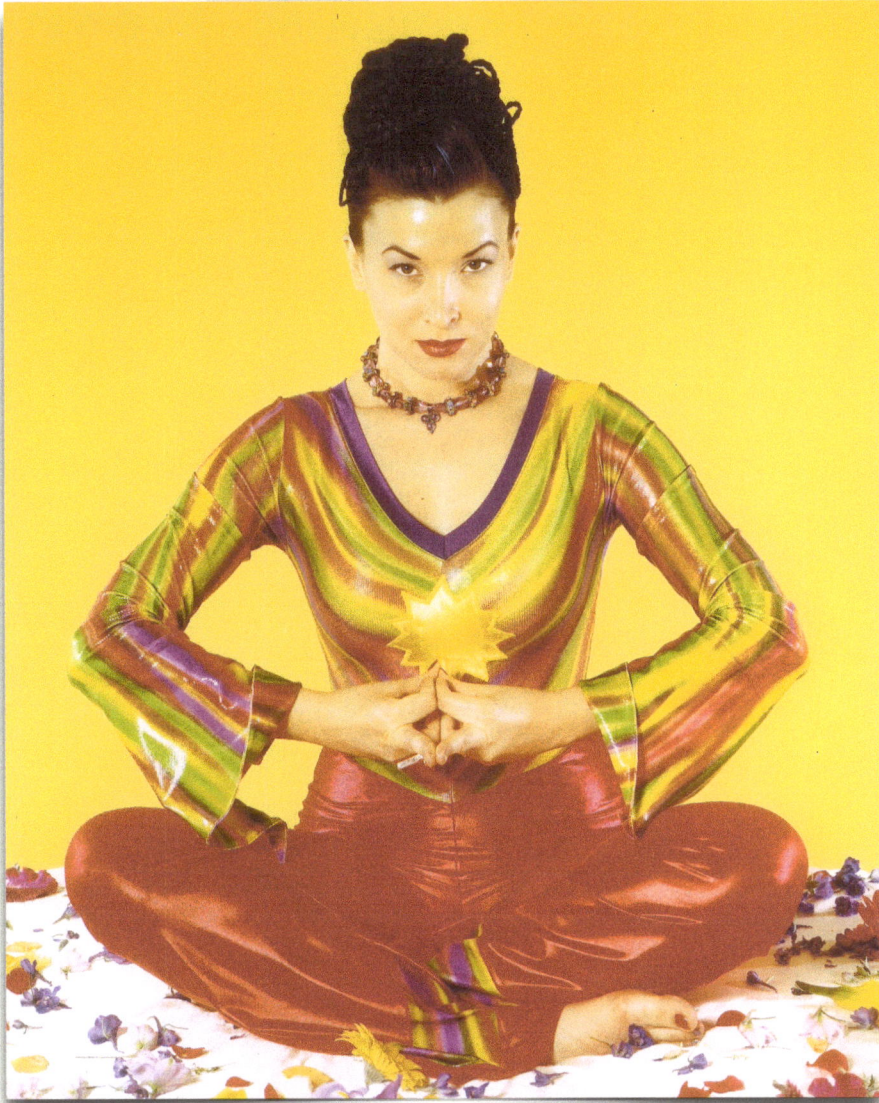

Sit with a straight spine and, with elbows bent, bring the hands up at the level of the navel. Bend the index fingers toward the palm and press them together along the second joint. Extend your middle fingers so that their finger pads are touching, pointing them away from your body. Curl the other fingers into your palm and touch the thumbs together at their tips, pointing toward you. Hold the mudra a few inches away from your body, elbows ad hands held at the same level.

BREATH: LONG, DEEP AND SLOW. Continue for a few minutes and concentrate.

MUDRA FOR DIMINISHING WORRIES

We all worry about something. Sometimes we worry out of habit, but there are times when we face truly difficult challenges. No matter what the magnitude of your problems, you can get a better perspective on them and take charge of your life with this mudra.

This mudra will connect the Saturn - middle fingers
for mental patience and reducing your worries.

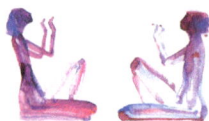

CHAKRA: Heart – 4
Throat – 5
Third Eye - 6

COLOR: Green, Blue, Indigo

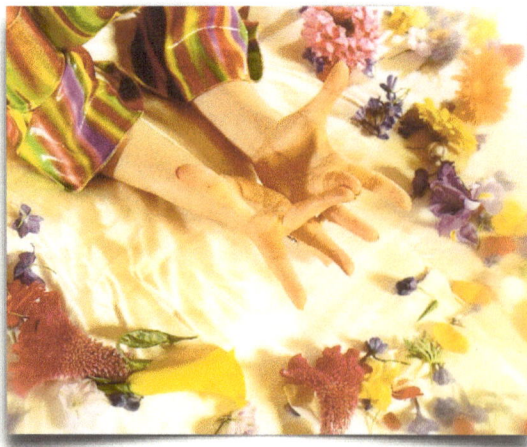

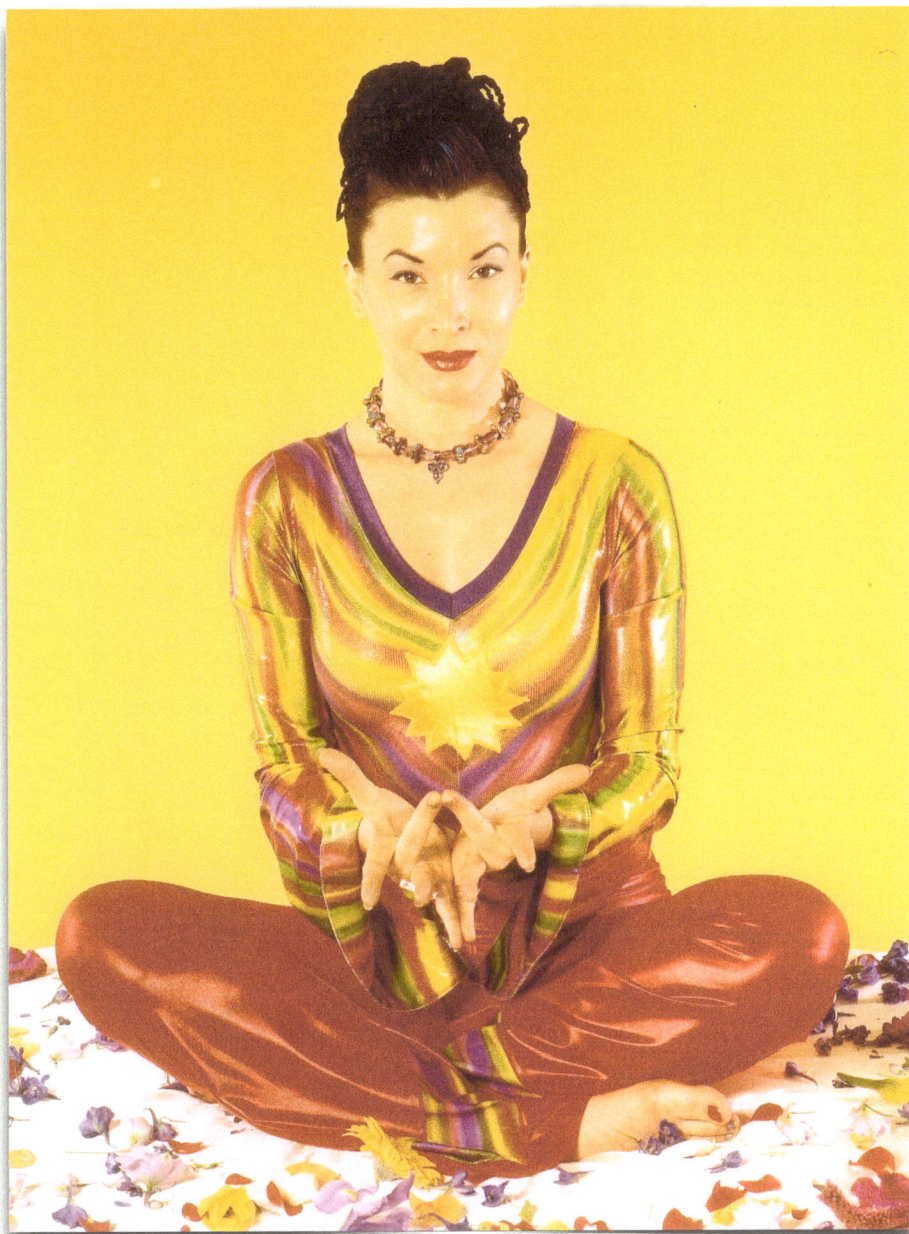

Sit with a straight back and bring your hands in front of your chest, palms facing up. The sides of the little fingers and inner sides of the palms are touching. Middle fingers are perpendicular to the palms, tips touching. Thumbs are extended away from the palms. Hold this mudra away from your chest. **BREATH:** LONG, DEEP AND SLOW. Continue for a few minutes and relax.

MUDRA FOR REMOVING DEPRESSION

For those times in life when everything seems bleak, if you can make an effort to do this mudra for only eleven minutes, your low feelings will diminish. Practice it once a day for a week and notice the difference. If your depression has lasted for two weeks, see your doctor or healthcare professional.

The power of this mudra will help cure the worst depression. The position of your arms, hands, and fingers will send healing and positive vibrations to your brain centers, affecting your glands, which will help you remove this condition.
You must practice for at least eleven minutes each time.

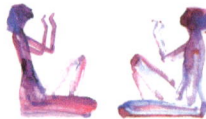

CHAKRA: Heart - 4
Throat – 5
Third Eye - 6
COLOR: Green, Blue, Indigo
MANTRA: HARI NAM SAT NAM, SAT NAM HARI NAM
~ God is Truth in Creation ~
Repeat mentally with each breath

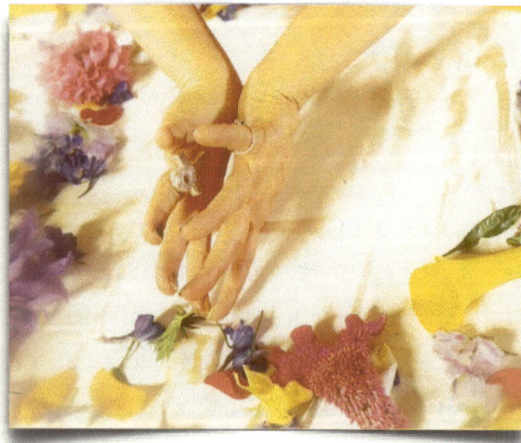

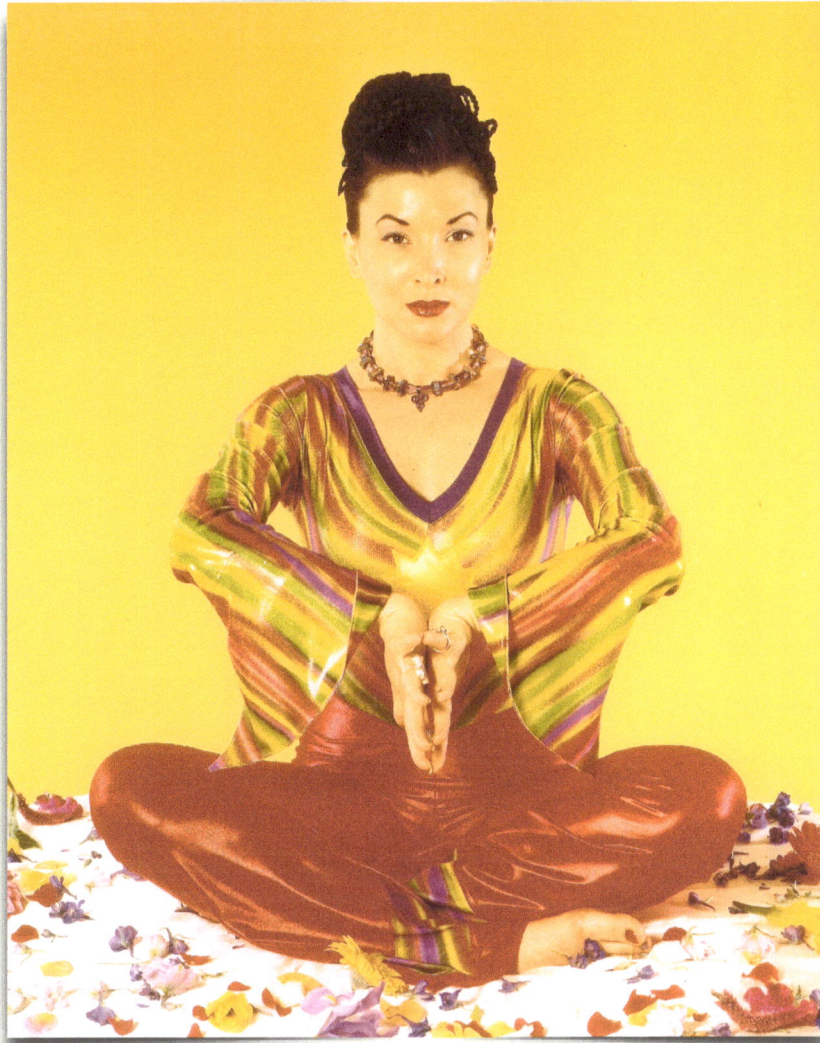

Sit with a straight spine. Stretch your arms in front of you, hands up at heart level. Put the backs of your hands together, with your fingers pointing away from your body, making sure that as many as possible knuckles touch. Your forearms are as parallel to the ground as possible, thumbs pointing down to the ground. This mudra creates a great deal of tension on the back part of your hands, but do not do this too long if you feel your muscles or tendons straining.

BREATH: LONG, DEEP AND SLOW. Continue for at least eleven minutes and feel the depression diminishing with each exhalation until it is gone.

MUDRA FOR SELF - CONFIDENCE

A positive mind, body, and spirit are necessary for fulfilling your life's desires. Daily practice of this mudra will change your life and make you so self-confident that you will inspire others.

The power of this mudra adjusts the energy of the perception centers
of your brain and improves your projection of positive energy.
It also prevents self - defeating thoughts and actions.

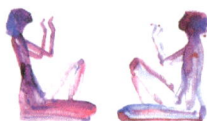

CHAKRA: Solar Plexus - 3
Third Eye - 6
COLOR: Yellow, Indigo
MANTRA: EK ONG KAR SAT GURU PRASAD
SAT GURU PRASAD EK ONG KAR
~ The Creator Is One That Dispels Darkness
and Illuminates Us by His Grace ~
Repeat mentally with each breath.

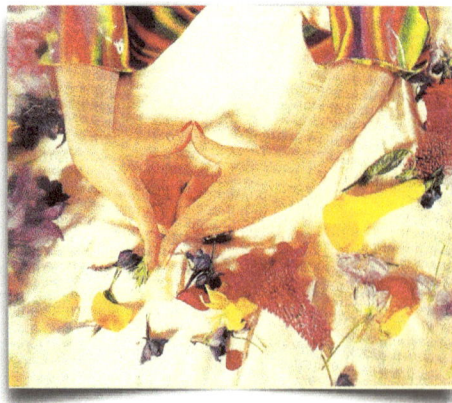

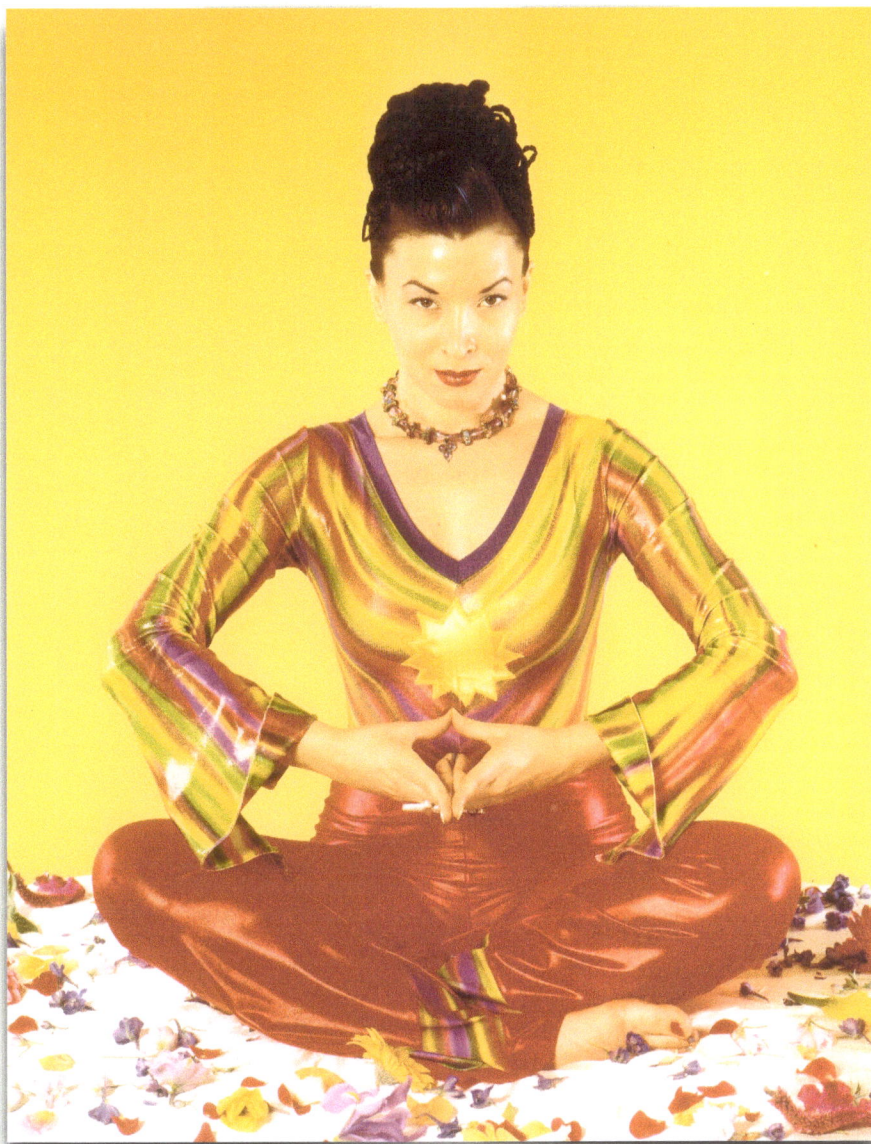

Sit comfortably with a straight spine. Lift your hands up to the level between your stomach and heart, elbows extended away from your body to the sides. Touch the middle knuckles of the last three fingers together. Point your index fingers out and away from your body, pads together. Point your thumbs back toward your chest as far as possible, touching each other from the last knuckle to the tip. Your thumbs are touching your body at the point of the solar plexus. **BREATH:** LOG, DEEP AND SLOW. Hold for a few minutes and relax.

MUDRA FOR RIGHT SPEECH

Right speech is one of the five precepts, or virtues, that the Buddha taught as important for the spiritual path. Clear communication is essential for our survival. "Think before you speak" is good advice, but sometimes we are prompted to make impulsive responses and statements that harm ourselves and others. This mudra is your key for better speech and control of emotions. It will help you say what you wish so you can get what you want. You will gain friends and not enemies.

This mudra will make what you say consistent with your true intentions.
It will also help you avoid saying things you don't mean.

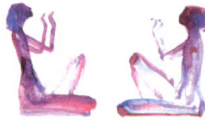

CHAKRA: Solar Plexus 3
Throat - 5
COLOR: Yellow, Blue
MANTRA: HAR DHAM HAR HAR
~ God Is the Creator ~
Repeat mentally with each breath

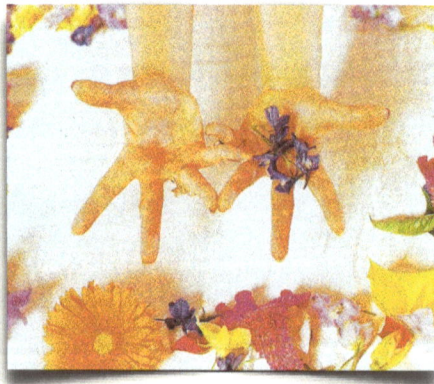

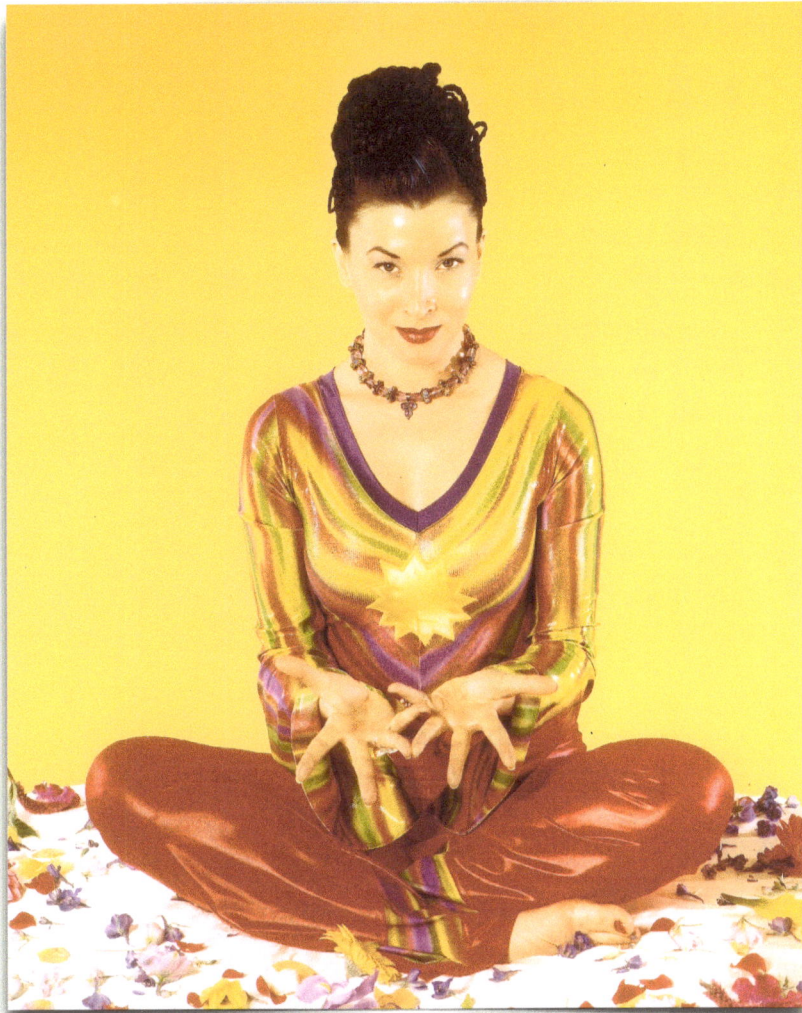

Sit with a straight spine. Relax your arms, keep your elbows at your sides, and bring your hands up in front of your stomach, palms open and flat, facing up. Spread your fingers gently and touch the tips of the ring fingers together, the right little finger is under the left little finger. Now concentrate and tense the thumb and the index fingers without moving the fingers. Hold for a few seconds and release. Now tense the thumb and the middle fingers, again without moving. Hold for a few seconds, and release.Next, tense the thumb and the ring fingers. Hold and release. Lastly, tense the thumb and little fingers, hold for a few seconds, and relax. Repeat the cycle reversing the little fingers and relax.

BREATH: LONG, DEEP AND SLOW.

MUDRA FOR UNBLOCKING THE SUBCONSCIOUS MIND

In our subconscious mind, we carry the memory and effects of positive and negative experiences. The energy of these negative memories – even if they are subconscious – can prevent us from reaching our true potential. You can tap into your subconscious memory, open it up, and clear it of these energy blockages with his mudra, which makes space for positive and powerful new energy flow. Then you can refocus your thoughts and activities on fulfilling your life's mission.

This mudra will aid in the process of self-evaluation and transformation by stimulating the Third Eye points with the thumbs and fingers.

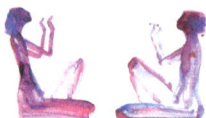

CHAKRA: Third Eye - 6
Crown - 7
COLOR: Indigo, Violet
MANTRA: ONG NAMO GURU DEV NAMO
~ I Bow to the Infinity of the Creator, I Call on the Infinite
Creative Consciousness and Divine Wisdom ~
Repeat mentally with each breath

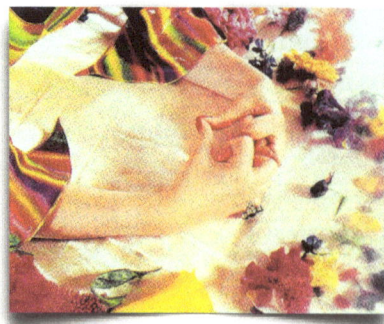

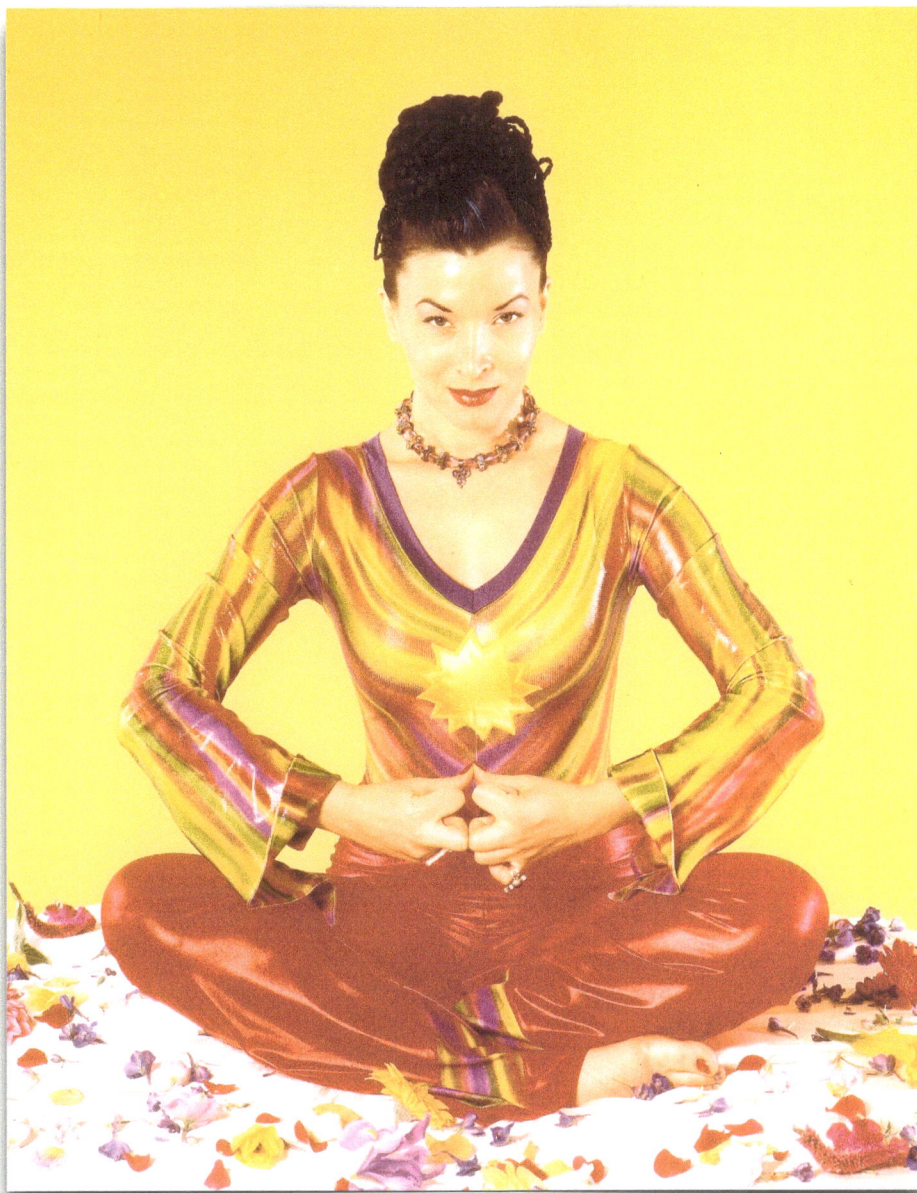

Sit with a straight spine. Relax and lift your arms up, out in front of you, elbows bent so your hands are in front of your stomach. Curl the fingers in so that the pads are touching the fleshy mounds at the base of the fingers. Thumb tips are together and the middle knuckles of the middle fingers are touching. No other fingers touch. Point your thumbs in a little toward the heart center. **BREATH:** LONG, DEEP AND SLOW. Concentrate on the warmth between the thumbs, continue for a few minutes and relax.

MUDRA FOR COMPASSION

Each of us is born into a different set of circumstances and environment. Some people seem luckier than others, so we must always remember to count our blessings and feel compassion for others less fortunate. You can never truly imagine someone else's situation unless you have gone through a similar experience. The practice of being nonjudgmental and compassionate in our hearts is key to progress on our spiritual path and to sending good energy throughout the Universe.

This mudra engages the heart center of compassion and the healing energy of the hands.
It increases the circulation of the blood to the brain,
clears the mind, and improves concentration.

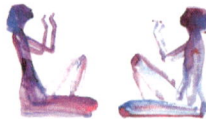

CHAKRA: Heart - 4

COLOR: Green

MANTRA: AKAL AKAL SIRI AKAL
~ Timeless Is the One Who Achieves Perfection of the Spirit ~
Repeat mentally with each breath.

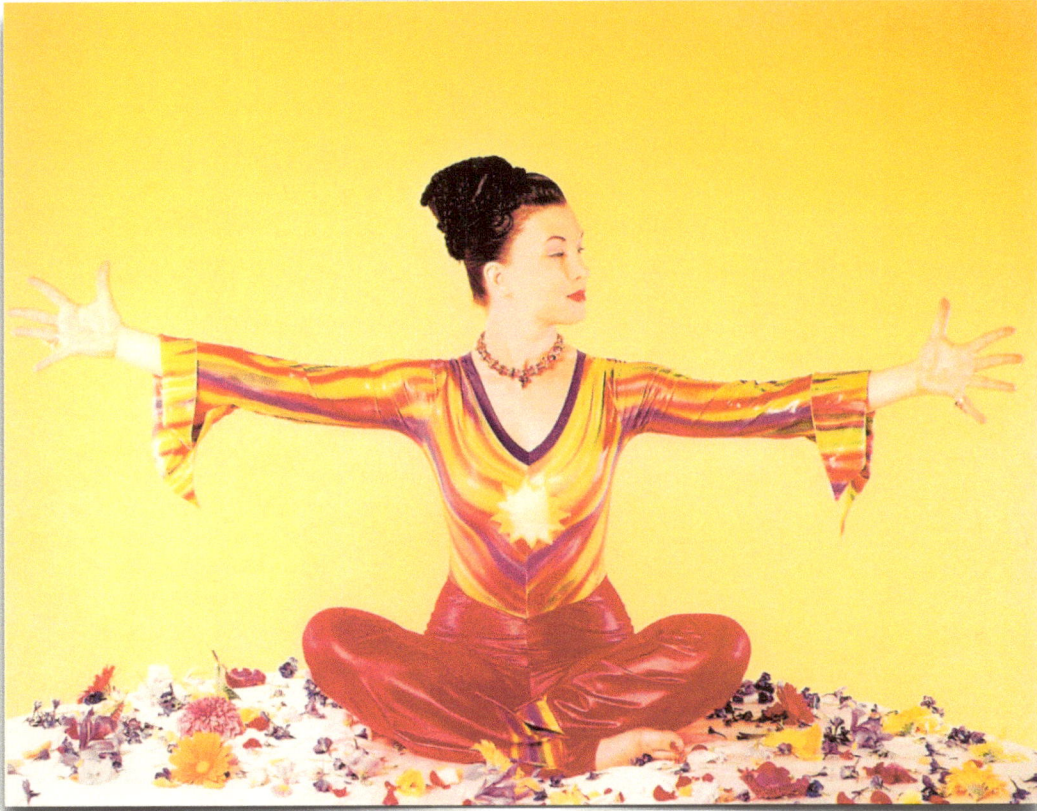

Sit with a straight spine. Extend your arms out to the sides parallel to the ground with the palms turned out front. Stretch out the fingers and hold them still. Turn your head to the right side and back to the center four times, then to the left side and back to the center four times. Continue for a few minutes and concentrate on your heart center. Be aware of the energy in your hands.

BREATH: INHALE LONG ONCE AS YOU MOVE YOUR HEAD TO THE RIGHT AND EXHALE LONG ONCE YOU MOVE YOUR HEAD BACK TO CENTER. REPEAT THE SAME FOR THE OTHER SIDE.

Relax and sit still for a few minutes.

THE SACRED MUDRA SEQUENCE
For Mental, Emotional and Energy Body Balance and Cleanse

This very specific mudra sequence is called Kirtan Kriya. It is an excellent and effective tool to cleanse your Auric field and bring the mental, physical and emotional body into a state of balance. The pituitary and pineal glands are stimulated, the negative thought patterns can be erased and a new balance is established.

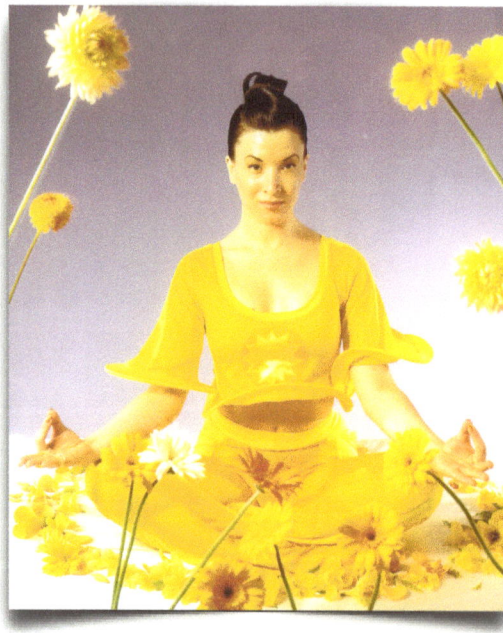

MANTRA:
SA TA NA MA
~ Infinity, Life, Death, Rebirth ~

Sit with a straight spine and rest the wrists on your knees. If possible stretch your elbows. Close your eyes and mentally focus on the area of the Third Eye. You will be connecting the thumb fingertips with other fingertips in a specific order sequence, while repeating the mantra.

TIMING:

THE MUDRA MANTRA SEQUENCE IS REPEATED AS FOLLOWS:

3 MINUTES IN NORMAL VOICE ~ awake state, earthly realm, the world

3 MINUTES IN LOUD WHISPER ~ longing to belong

6 MINUTES IN SILENCE ~ divine infinity

3 MINUTES IN LOUD WHISPER

3 MINUTES IN NORMAL VOICE VOLUME

These three modes of chanting relate to three levels of meditation:
With regular practice extend each segment to 5 min. and silence to 10 min.
Upon completion of this meditation sequence, deeply inhale and exhale,
stretch your arms up, spread your fingers, breathe long, deep and relax.

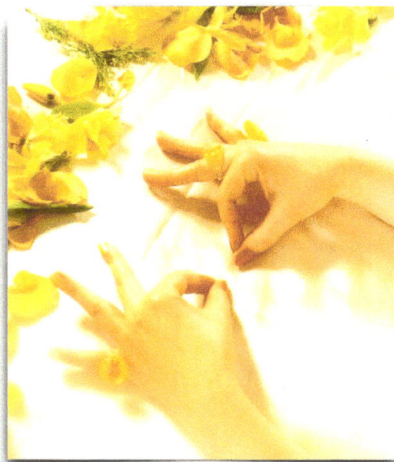

FIRST POSITION:
Connect and press together the thumbs
and index fingers while chanting: **SA**

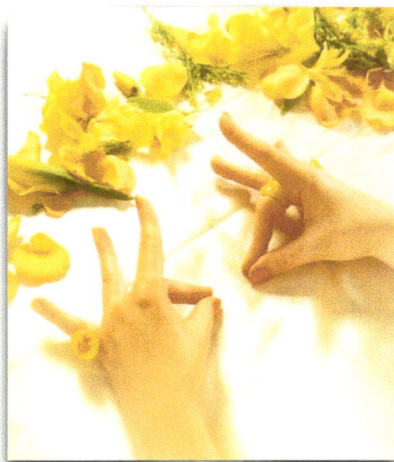

SECOND POSITION:
Connect and press together the thumbs
and middle fingers while chanting: **TA**

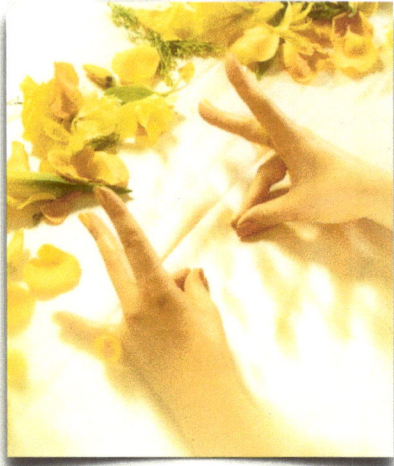

THIRD POSITION:
Connect and press together the thumbs and ring fingers while chanting: **NA**

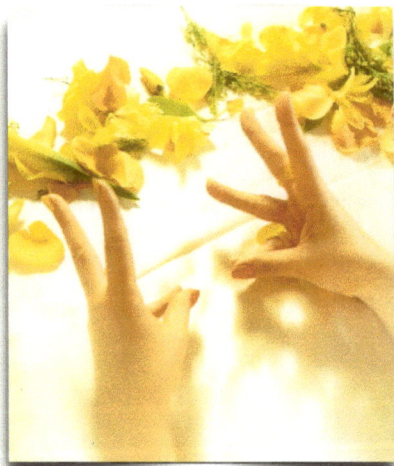

FOURTH POSITION:
Connect and press together the thumbs and ring fingers while chanting: **MA**

MUDRA INDEX

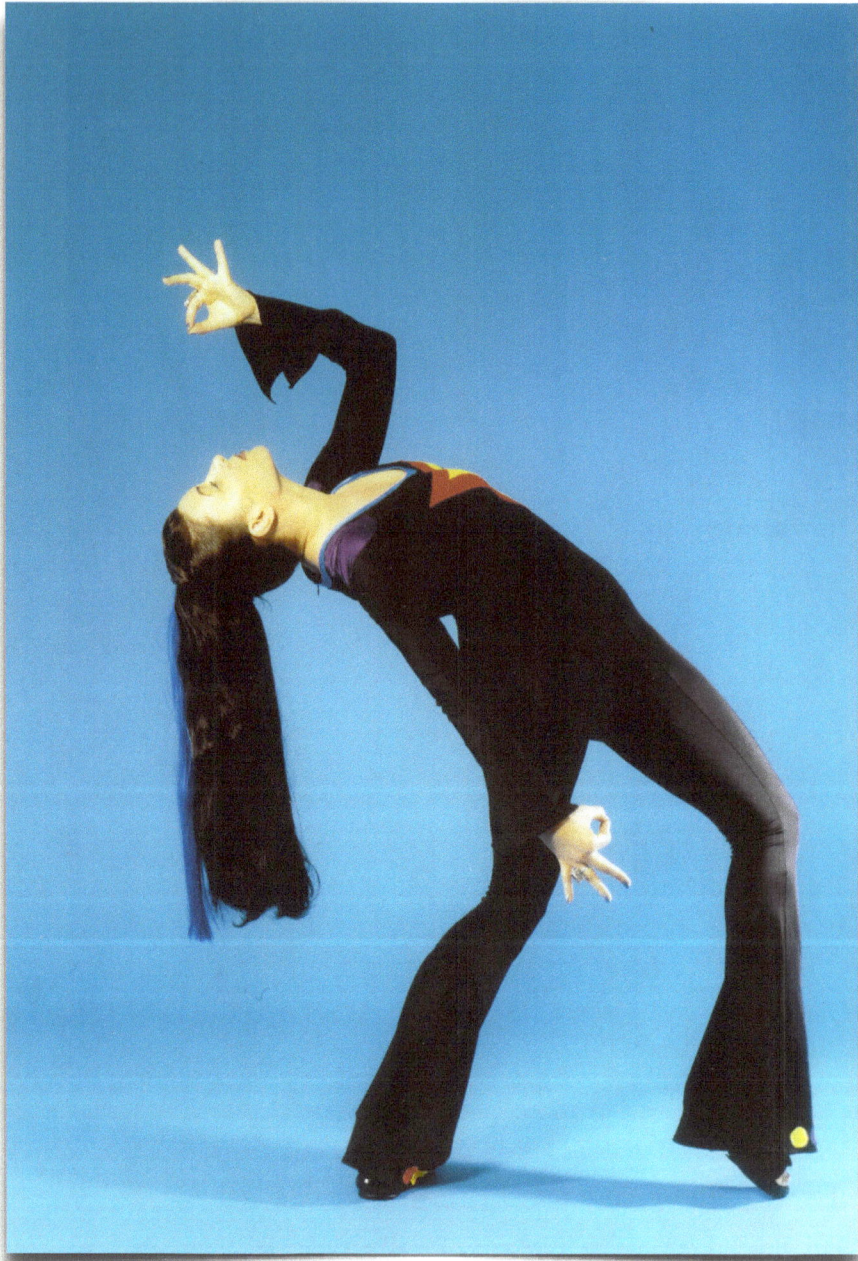

ABOUT THE AUTHOR

SABRINA MESKO   Ph.D.H. is a recognized Mudra authority and International and Los Angeles Times bestselling author of the timeless classic *Healing Mudras - Yoga for your Hands* translated into fourteen languages, as well as twenty other books on Mudras, Mudra Therapy, Mudras and Astrology, and meditation techniques.

Sabrina was born in Europe where she became a classical ballerina at an early age. In her teens she moved to New York and became a principal Broadway dancer and singer who turned to yoga to heal a back injury. She studied with Master Guru Maya, healing breath techniques with Master Sri Sri Ravi Shankar and completed a four-year study of Paramahansa Yogananda's Kriya Yoga technique. She graduated from the internationally known Yoga College of India and became a certified yoga therapist. An immense interest and study of powerful hand gestures - Mudras, led Sabrina to the world's only Master of White Tantric Yoga, Yogi Bhajan, who entrusted her with the sacred Mudra - hand yoga techniques giving her the responsibility to spread this ancient and powerful knowledge worldwide. She studied with him privately under his personal mentorship and guidance, and continues to teach Mudra techniques as taught by him.

Sabrina holds a Bachelors Degree in Sensory Approaches to Healing, a Masters in Holistic Science, and a Doctorate in Ancient and Modern Approaches to Healing from the American Institute of Holistic Theology. She is board certified from the American Alternative medical Association and American Holistic Health Association.

She has been featured in media outlets such as The Los Angeles Times, CNBC News, Cosmopolitan, the cover of London Times Lifestyle, The Discovery Channel documentary on Hands, W magazine, First for Women, Health, WebMD, Daily News, Focus, Yoga Journal, Australian Women's weekly, Blend, Daily Breeze, New Age, the Roseanne Show and various international live television programs. Her articles have been published in world-wide publications. She hosted her own weekly TV show educating about health, well-being and complementary medicine. She is an executive member of the World Yoga Council and has led numerous international Yoga Therapy educational programs. She directed and produced her interactive double DVD titled *Chakra Mudras* - a Visionary awards finalist. Sabrina also created award winning international Spa and Wellness Centers and is a motivational keynote conference speaker addressing large audiences all over the world. Sabrina recently launched Arnica Press, a boutique Book Publishing House. Her mission is to discover, mentor, nurture and publish unique authors with a meaningful message, that may otherwise not have an opportunity to be heard.

She is the founder of MUDRA MASTERY ™ the world's only online Mudra Teacher and Mudra Therapy Education, Certification, and Mentorship program, with her certified graduates and therapists spreading these ancient teachings in over 26 countries around the world.

WWW.SABRINAMESKO.COM

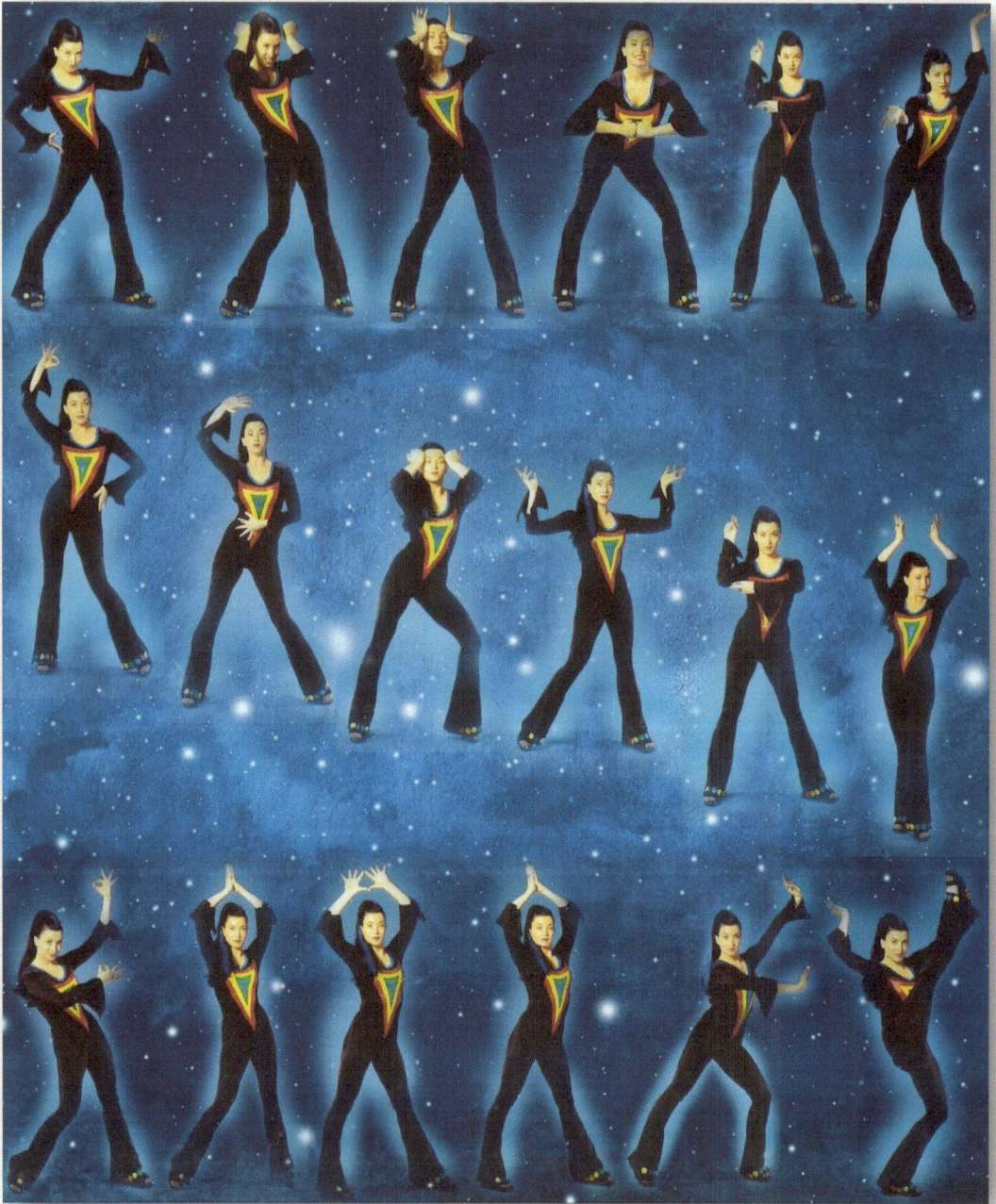

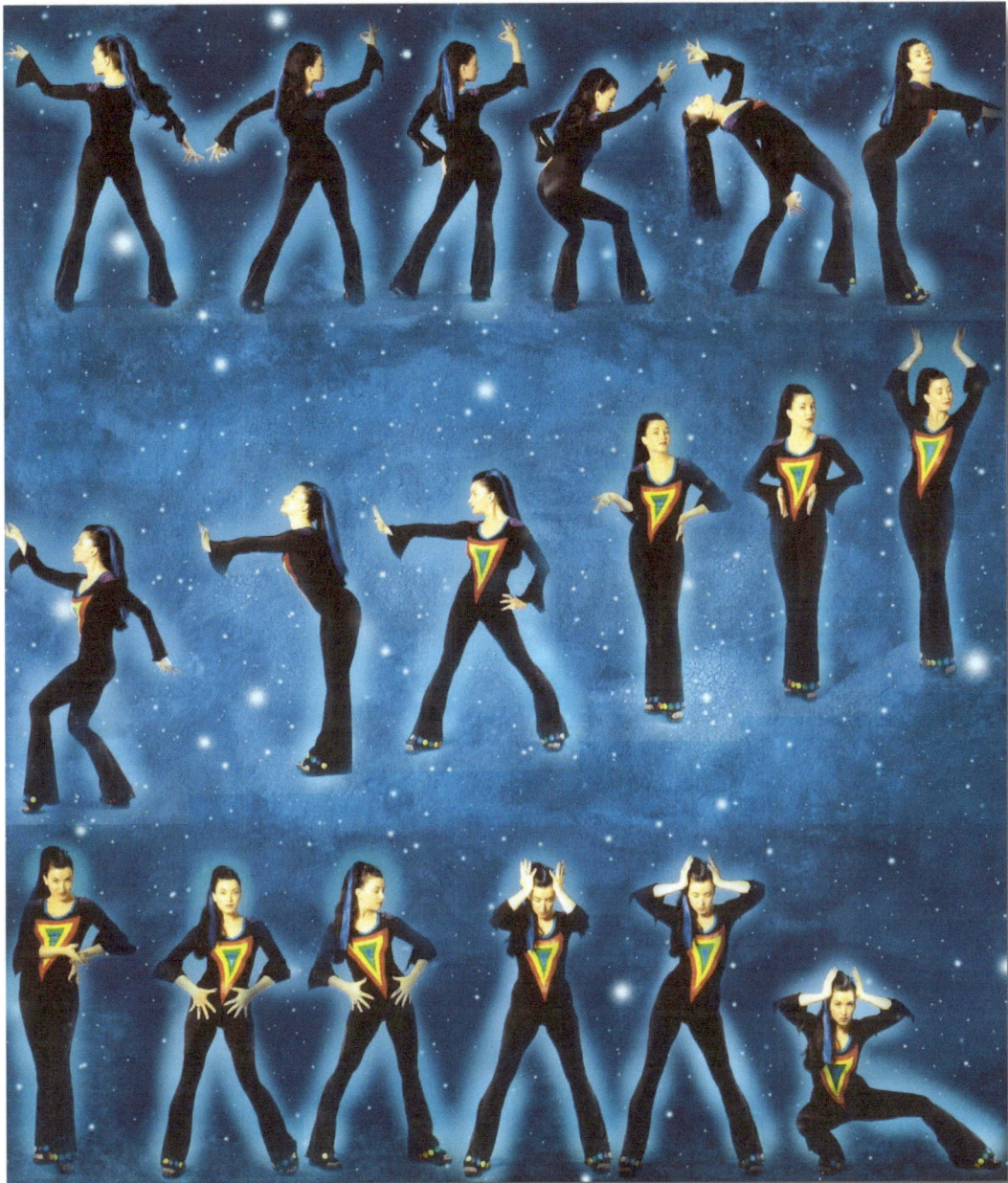

www.ingramcontent.com/pod-product-compliance
Lightning Source LLC
Chambersburg PA
CBHW060805270326
41927CB00002B/59